T0336875

A VOYAGE INTO THE HUMAN MIND

# A FRIEND IN ME EMOTION LESS RELATIONSHIP

## PSYCHOLOGIST. PREETI PANDIT

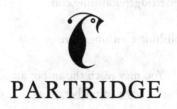

PARTRIDGE

**To order additional copies of this book, contact**
Toll Free 800 101 2657 (Singapore)
Toll Free 1 800 81 7340 (Malaysia)
orders.singapore@partridgepublishing.com

www.partridgepublishing.com/singapore

You may reach the author at:
www.mindtherapy.sg

Dr Preeti Pandit is a practising psychologist, counsellor, and psychotherapist based in Singapore. She has her independent practice, certified by Singapore Association for Counselling (SAC) and affilated to Centre for Complementary and Alternative Medicine (CCAM). She is the wind beneath the wings of her family-owned Sandpiper Hotels in Singapore and Kuala Lumpur. She has also been nominated as one of the Top 50 Most Influential Women in Singapore.

A very impressive résumé, but these credentials are like a drop in her ocean of talent, experiences, and achievements.

Born in India, Dr Preeti completed her basic education in Bhopal, India, and graduated from Agra, India. She is the epitome of beauty with brains. While she won accolades in academics during her growing years, she also won the Miss Bhopal India beauty contest in her teens. She pursued her postgraduate degree and did her research from Nimhans (National Institute of Mental Health and Neurosciences) in Bangalore, India, followed by a special course on mental health from Rice University in Houston, USA. She completed the research for her PhD but could not complete the process since she had to come back from the United States for family reasons.

She developed a penchant for helping people very early in her life, so becoming a therapist was a very natural extension of her passion. Her ability to make the other person feel wanted, her relentless drive to create a shift in people's lives, and her willingness to experiment endeared her to every client who worked with her.

The mother of one of her clients said, 'I cannot forget that you literally walked with me in my moments of despair. You gave me hope that my child can be helped. Even as I type, my eyes swell with tears and flow down my cheeks. No amount of money can be paid for this kindness of yours.'

Another client had this to say: 'The therapy was a great release for me. There was good relief, and with it came lots of healing, mind space, change in perspective of my problems, and a realignment of their priorities in life. The world is a big place. Slowly and surely, I have hope and light in my life again.'

Yet another client said, 'My experience with psychotherapy has been truly rewarding. It has helped me walk out of darkness, and I find myself continually improving still, every day. With your guidance, I have gone from crying every day and being needy to being healthy and independent. Through you, I have been able to release anger, worry, fear, grief, and guilt and experience compassion, wisdom, light, and love.'

Dr Pandit has a very calm persona and has a reassuring presence about her, but what makes her effective is her approach.

Dr Pandit says, 'I decide my course of action based on the client and the situation. In fact, I seem to be blessed with a strange intuition which guides me on the next steps.' She can be very experimental with her therapies, which is probably the reason for her effectiveness. She is strongly against her clients taking any form of medication. Rather, she believes in the restoration of the natural balance between the body and mind as the solution to most ailments.

Dr Pandit uses self-projection techniques, where one must identify the talents which lie dormant in the self. For example, you may be good at creative arts, such as dance, painting, music, or any other form which enhances self-recognition and self-esteem. During childhood, parents must look out for these seeds and provide nourishment, training, and encouragement. Later in life, one has to pursue these interests on his or her own. Self-projection is considered one of the most profound and subtle ways of human psychological processes and is extremely difficult to work with. This is because the skills backing this process are hidden. It's creative only when projected to the outside world. Improving self-projection reduces anxiety by providing an expression to these creative and unconscious impulses or desires without the conscious mind recognising them.

Apart from standard techniques of psychotherapy, Dr Pandit recommends 'Book therapy' as a therapeutic measure for healing patients who are attempting to recover from traumas. Book therapy uses stories and drawings to process difficult emotions. She believes that stories and symbolic images can help people connect to their deeper feelings that they find difficult to talk about. Accordingly, she uses a combination of face-to-face counselling and Book therapy to help patients move past the emotional issues that keep them stuck.

When it comes to relationships, she has also used 'reality therapy', which teaches couples how to manage wants and needs in a relationship. It can help a couple to face the realities of situations, towards restoring harmony in their marriage.

Dr Pandit is also not averse to using 'behaviour therapy' to cure addictions. This therapy is based on experimentally derived principles of learning, which are systematically applied to help people change their maladaptive behaviour. It deals with clients' current problems and the factors influencing them, as opposed to an analysis of possible historical factors. Behaviour therapy also emphasises the self-control approach, in which clients learn self-management strategies. Therapists frequently train clients to initiate, conduct, and evaluate their own therapy.

Another therapy that she commonly uses is 'swim therapy'. Herself an accomplished swimmer and scuba diver, she uses this therapy as a technique for confidence building, especially if the person is a nonswimmer, is afraid of water (aquaphobia), or even has a fear of bathing (ablutophobia). She believes that a swimming pool is an excellent location where the swimmer goes through multiple steps to restore his or her confidence and trains the mind's every moment. Dr Pandit says, 'For a swimmer in therapy, every stroke is a choice between going ahead and sinking. As he becomes deft in moving ahead, overcoming fear becomes a habit which moulds his character and finally makes the person succeed in all adverse situations against any phobia.'

Dr Pandit is also an accomplished painter. She started with oil paintings in her early teens and became proficient in the Chhattisgarhi form during her stay in Bhopal. One of the paintings close to her heart is an oil painting of Umar Khayyam and Mirza Ghalib, which she completed in ninth grade. Even without any formal training, she would win a prize in almost every competition that she took part in. With her exposure to different cultures, she slowly graduated to other art forms. During her stay in Moscow, she learnt the Russian form of painting called *fidoski,* and her paintings were even displayed in an exhibition at the Moscow Art Museum. She learnt the nuances of *palekh* painting, where one needs to paint miniatures under a lens. The Singapore government has featured her paintings in a coffee table book.

She says, 'Art is a therapy for me. It detoxifies me after my intense sessions.' This realisation prompted her to use art as a therapy for her clients. Art psychotherapy is a means of symbolic communication. It emphasises the elements—like drawings, paintings, and other artistic expressions—as being helpful in communicating issues, emotions, and resolving internal conflicts. From an artist's perspective, indulgence in art is seen as an opportunity to express oneself imaginatively, authentically, and spontaneously. It is considered to be an experience that, over time, can lead to personal fulfilment.

Due to her husband's work, she got the opportunity to visit and stay in many countries. Many of these experiences form part of this book. Apart from understanding cultures, she left her indelible mark wherever she lived.

During her eight years in Myanmar, Dr Pandit was a guest lecturer of psychology at Dagon University. She even helped the university set up a psychology lab. Her work rewarded her with a special invitation from the first lady of India at that time, Mrs Usha Narayanan, the wife of the then President Mr K. R. Narayanan. The first lady was Burmese, and her relatives in Myanmar gave a wonderful description about Dr Pandit to their illustrious family member. Along with having an opportunity to interact with senior government ministers, she also had the privilege to meet Ms Aung San Suu Kyi. These interactions brought her into the limelight and presented her with an opportunity to demonstrate her leadership skills as the president of the International Charity Group in Myanmar. For someone who dabbled in poetry during her childhood, she also received in Myanmar the chance to express herself through her writings in the United Nations Women's Association magazine.

During her stay in Cuba, she met many ministers and provided her views on policies regarding mental health. She had the privilege to meet President Fidel Castro, an interaction she still cherishes.

She has always wanted to make a positive difference in the lives of people. Seeing the pitiable condition of street children in Myanmar, she set up an orphanage home, where she housed eighteen to twenty children, taking care of their food, medicines, and clothing. Her son and daughter would spend some time with the children and teach English, maths, and computers. She urged her husband's company to donate their old stationery and computers to the orphanage. Before she moved out of the country, she even ensured that some of the orphaned boys got a job in her husband's company and gifted a few girls with sewing machines, which would help them make a living.

She credits her calm persona to Vipassana meditation, of which she is an ardent follower. Having personally met the renowned Mr Goenka, the founder of Vipassana centres in India and abroad, she has attended around eight retreats, including one at the Alps in Switzerland, and has even recommended this life-enhancing experience to some of her clients.

She is very meticulous about things, and with her eye for detail and understanding of colours, she has personally monitored the design of her hotels. The Sandpiper logo is her creation, and she can often be found on her favourite couch opposite the huge logo in the hotel lobby.

She now lives in Singapore with her husband and son. She has been honoured with an award for being the symbol of the aspirational and modern woman by Doyenne Singapore. Her husband is an astute businessman who manages the hotel chain, and her son Graduated from Switzerland, is a budding entrepreneur who is making his presence felt in the business world. Her daughter is Bio medical Engineer from Harvard and Tuffs USA, Director of Abbott, now married.

Some of Dr Pandit's thoughts and ideas are published in the blog www.pardeshipulse.com/blogdir.

# FOREWORD

Shri O. P. Sarbhoy
MA (economics), MA (SW), LLB
retired director (P&A) of National Hydroelectric Power
Corporation Ltd., India
father of the author

I am glad to know that my daughter, Preeti Pandit, who is a practising clinical psychologist and an accredited counsellor in Singapore, has written this book on psychosocial problems of living. The book is a graphic narrative of her own life experience, combined with the knowledge gained from actual cases that she has dealt with as a counsellor. In this context, I consider it appropriate to mention some of her traits that were noticed during her growing years, which, I believe, were the earliest indication of her nature.

Destiny, it is said, is not so much a matter of fate as it is of the choices one makes in life. Every moment we are making a choice of what we do or don't do from amongst the many options available. What makes the difference is the choice made, its outcome, and the determination to hold on to the same with responsibility. Preeti displayed a distinct sense of choice at every stage of her life. Even as a child, just six months old, she would quickly grab a particular pink frock and would cry to wear it instead of any other. This trend was visible all through her life, whether it was the choice of her life partner or her career.

Intrinsic in her nature was a keen desire to learn and do things that could bring her laurels and eventually wider acceptance in society. Perhaps this was the driving force that inspired her to take up oil painting with a passion. She would paint a large canvas all night long, until it was presentable. Later, when in Moscow, where she stayed for about three years, she learnt mini lacquer painting and did many small plates, which she gifted to friends and relatives. Her paintings started as a hobby when she was in school. Even without any formal training, her paintings were judged as prize winners at college-level competitions. This gave her a great measure of self-confidence and courage to take up challenging tasks in life.

Her research paper on the relationship between self-esteem and performance in secondary school children, undertaken as a fulfilment of her MPhil, enhanced her own conviction in building up self-esteem and the ability to go out and engage in social activities with success.

Her social skills came to the fore while in Moscow, where she successfully brought together isolated womenfolk of expatriated and diplomatic staff into a closely-knit ladies' social club. She played a pivotal role in the club and organised many activities. This approach she repeated in Yangon (Myanmar), where she lived for almost five years.

The above social activities made it easier for her to move into the elite social circles while giving her husband social support in his business wherever he was posted.

With her husband deciding to take premature retirement and settle down in Singapore, she established her psychological counselling clinic and in a short span of time attained popularity.

With her unflinching support, her husband decided to enter the hotel business. In a short duration, they have put up two hotels—one in Singapore and the other in Kuala Lumpur (Malaysia) under the banner of Sandpiper Hotels.

Her enterprising nature has been recognised by the Singapore government, for which she was formally honoured and listed in the book *Doyen of Singapore.*

I wish this book all success and wide acceptance.

\*\*\*

Dr Ira Saxena
Saxena.ira@gmail.com
Author and psychologist, India; convener, Book Therapy Project

**A Friendly Touch**

Care, concern, and compassion are some of the distinctive features of a friend, a well-wisher, a healer. They magnetise a distressed person in search of a buddy to unburden the strains of life situations, to be relieved and alleviated of stress. A friendly touch becomes a curative touch, spreading the balm of silent tranquillity over the clamour of conflicts, eventually restoring stability and inner peace.

Care is an attitude in the personality of Preeti Pandit, the author of this book, a successful psychological counsellor, actually a healer, augmenting her professional style. Her concern for the patient awakens every little observation in her analysis, and the force of her fervent compassion supersedes a clinical approach in dealing with her patients. Over and above, I would ascribe the X factor in her mental make-up, an out-of-the-ordinary sensitivity, predominantly reaching to delve the core of the incongruity. A natural friend in her dominates the patient, the therapy session, all, ensuring solace and promising total confidentiality. Only the spirit of a true friend for all times towers above for all those in need.

In the troubled waters of day-to-day existence, there is hardly anyone who does not undergo situations of anxiety, depression from demanding circumstances, stressful relationships, and struggles of coping with troubles and tribulations. Psychotherapy aims to improve a person's well-being, to resolve or mitigate antisocial attitudes, distressing behaviours, compulsive thoughts, and discordant emotions, enabling social skills and normal social interaction. Distressing conditions caused by loss, failure, deficits, shortfalls, financial crises, and broken relationships block the smooth flow of life for adults as children could suffer challenges from loss, family discord, peer pressure, expectations of performance, and so on, threatening a surge of social conundrums along with maturational apprehensions. Such anxieties would naturally be debilitating to the adult or the child alike, intensifying pressures upon the troubled soul.

While people around may be supportive, they can never be so in the same way as the professional therapist, who is familiar with the processes and procedures to arrive quickly at the source of the conflicts and determine the appropriate track for reinstating normal health.

Each chapter in this book reveals some special aspects of personal and extramarital relations—its grip and predicaments, children's strains and worries, and impaired values among children—reinforcing improved communication skills with the child and the influence of stresses and depression upon the role of a value system in the child's world, as well as in adult life. The book references the personal experiences of the author in her practice as a counsellor, which, interestingly, authenticate the author's unique procedures and philosophies.

*A Friend in Me, Emotional Relationship* provides a panorama of the experience of Preeti, who has jumped conventional boundaries of psychological healing, combining it with the unique application of features like meditation and book therapy techniques.

The realities of people in society and the expanse of thought-provoking issues in this book distinguish it as an exceptionally motivating read any day, anywhere, anytime.

In the pages, a real friend comes around to stay with you.

***

Dr V. P. Nair, MBBS, MRCP, FRCP (London, Edinburgh, and Ireland)
FAMS (cardiology), FESC (France), FCCP, FACC, and FSCAI (USA)
consultant cardiologist, Mount Elizabeth Medical Centre, Singapore

A fast-paced lifestyle crammed with personal commitments and work deadlines is taking a toll on our physical and mental health. People who are anxious or depressed may turn to a general practitioner, social worker, psychologist, or psychiatrist for counselling and therapy. Psychiatry and psychology are overlapping professions. Their area of expertise is the mind and the way it affects behaviour and well-being. They often work together to prevent, diagnose, and treat mental illness.

Consultant psychologist Dr Preeti Pandit, the author of the book *A Friend in Me*, has extensive experience in the analysis of the human mind and in identifying the underlying mental issues to restore happiness and harmony in the individual, family, and society.

In her book, she has illustrated a few interesting and informative cases of her own. Moreover, she has looked deeper into certain relationships to discover how a crack in these relationships may lead to depression, anxiety, and a sense of doom. This book will help us to realise hope and accomplishment.

\*\*\*

Dr Ajit Saxena
pioneer, urology robotic surgery
MS (Delhi), FRCS (Edinburgh), FICS, MNAMS (urology), diploma in urology (London)
senior consultant urologist and andrologist, Indraprastha Apollo Hospitals

It is with a sense of pride that I write this foreword. I have seen Preeti grow up since her childhood. From a shy little girl, she has matured into a multitalented lady. Her experience in various countries, including Nepal, Russia, China, Burma, the United States, Malaysia, and now Singapore, gives her invaluable in-depth knowledge of the human psyche.

With such vast experience, she has been invited as a visiting lecturer of psychology to such prestigious institutions as the Hartford Institute of Management (Central Queensland University, Australia) and the Singapore Institute of Management. She has conducted training programs in corporate offices in Singapore and is affiliated with the Singapore Quality Institute (SQI), Lee Community College.

A charming lady with over thirty years of work and academic experience, Preeti has been much sought after to write for many magazines and newsletters. She also has a number of academic publications.

With increasing technology and globalisation, there is also an increasing identity crisis. This book addresses family issues, including self-realisation and child upbringing. This book is a must for the expectant mother, as it is for retired persons staring into the future.

I wish Preeti all the success and hope that she continues to write on such relevant topics as those in this book.

# PREFACE

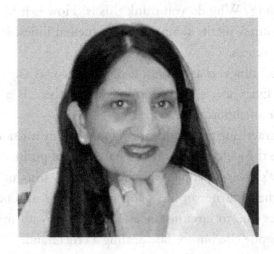

When you are joyous, look deep into your heart and you shall find it is only that which has given you sorrow that is giving you joy. When you are sorrowful look again in your heart, and you shall see that in truth you are weeping for that which has been your delight.
—Khalil Gibran www.brainyquote.com/quotes/khalil_gibran_121554

When you have an excruciating headache, you go to a doctor. The doctor understands the symptoms and diagnoses the cause. The doctor may either order more tests or give you a prescription of medicines. Your school or company gives you days off to recuperate from your illness, and most people are even sympathetic to your plight.

However, instead of a headache, what if you are having constant panic attacks? Due to the societal stigma, you don't go to the psychotherapist because you're worried. *What will people say?* When things get so out of hand that it starts affecting your normal life, you decide to seek help. However, everyone from your boss to your friends is telling you to 'suck it up' and 'just keep smiling'. Why do you think this is? How is it fair that a physical illness merits sympathy but a mental illness is looked at as a weakness?

Mental illness is as serious, if not more so, as any physical ailment. Everyone is born normal, unless there is a genetic reason for an abnormality.

As a practising psychotherapist, I make it my mission in life to change this perception and be a harbinger of positive change in people's lives—people who have strayed into unknown areas in their journey of life, people who have lost touch with themselves due to circumstances, and people who may have been someone else but for fate dealing a cruel hand.

Relationships are the crux of society as we have shaped it, such as the relationships between a mother and a child, between two friends, or between siblings. The imbalance in these relationships can create a long-lasting impact on one's psyche. This book will delve deeper into certain relationships and examine how a crack in them can be one of the causes of mental illnesses, such as depression, anxiety, and an overall sense of doom.

My experiences have also made me realise that the foundation of who we become in our adult lives is laid during our childhood. The environments, behaviours, and situations that a child is exposed to will determine, to a large extent, the kind of personality that is developed in later stages of life. A case in point is Mr Narendra Modi, the prime minister of India, who had a very humble childhood which made him determined and resilient, which is the hallmark of his personality today. On the other hand, his political opponent Mr Rahul Gandhi had a protected childhood, and his rise in the political party that he belongs to happened as an entitlement. His perceived lack of focus and lack of will to fight against all odds may be the effect of these privileges. The great Singapore leader Lee Kuan Yew experienced many hardships during his growing years due to the Japanese occupation, which influenced his political decisions.

During the last thirty years, my husband's work has taken the family to countries like Nepal, Cuba, Russia, and Myanmar. During all these years, I had the privilege to understand different cultures, spend time with my idols, work with local people, and make a difference in their lives. Life has gifted me with an eye for seeing things beyond what they are. Life has allowed me to meet lovely people and add value to their lives while enriching mine. I feel enriched, and I feel that it is time to share this bounty with the world. While I do receive appreciative emails from many of my clients, I feel indebted to each one of them for they have given me a new perspective to life.

In this book, I share my interactions with some special people who touched my life while I created a shift in theirs. My purpose is to showcase the fact that there is nothing wrong with sharing your inward and bottled-up feelings if it helps you move ahead and achieve your purpose in life.

This book will take a reader through encouraging interpersonal learning, questioning personal effectiveness, creating self-awareness, and examining 'criteria of fidelity of conscience'. When the distortion between what a person wants to communicate and what the other person understands is large, then individual effectiveness is low. It has taken me a journey of thirty years to awaken my feelings to help others. All I knew was my desire to understand people—what they think, why they behave in a certain way, and why different individuals react differently in the same situation.

This book is my way of giving to the world what I have received from it in abundance.

**Visit http://http://www.mindtherapy.sg/**

# CHAPTER 1

# THE CUBAN DIARIES

## 1

The month of November brings a lot of rain to Singapore. Humidity increases, and everything is wet and sticky. I prefer the summer months, when everything is bright and even the most mundane tasks seem welcoming.

It does feel depressing when lying on the bed—you get a glimpse of the dark grey sky through the little gap in the curtains, and you hear the constant drizzle making a seemingly never-ending sound as the drops of rain, slanted due to the light breeze, fall on the windowpane. Today was one such day. It did not help that I had only one therapy session to keep myself occupied. I finished the session and headed straight to the hotel. The sound of pleasing music, which I instantly recognised as the selection of Beethoven classics that I had ordered some days earlier, gave me an instant energy boost.

Our family owns the Sandpiper group of hotels, which has branches in Singapore and Malaysia. The lovely Michelle was at the reception desk, and she gave a warm smile while greeting me.

'Good evening, ma'am,' she said with a gentle bow of her head.

I reciprocated warmly. 'Very good evening, Michelle. How are you today?'

'Very well, ma'am,' she responded with her smile intact.

Michelle had joined the hotel a couple of weeks ago, and I was instantly drawn to her smile. I walked to the lounge and sat on my favourite couch right in front of the big Sandpiper logo.

'Ma'am, can I get a drink for you?' Michelle enquired from behind the reception.

My mood was already better just by being there, but who could refuse a nice cup of Darjeeling tea?

'Could you ask for some tea please?' I answered.

As she picked up the house telephone to place the order, my attention was drawn to the television across the room from where I was sitting. CNN was broadcasting the news. While the presenter was sharing some facts about the world economy, my eyes were riveted to the bottom of the screen and the scrolling message 'Fidel Castro dead'.

I blinked a few times to confirm that I was indeed reading the message correctly, and there it was again.

Since I could not increase the volume of the television in the lobby, I asked Michelle to give me the key to one of the rooms which we would always keep as an emergency spare for any special guest whom we might need to accommodate. My mind was racing as I took the elevator to the second floor and opened room 210.

I switched on the television, and it seemed like an eternity before it came on. I browsed through the channel list before I found CNN.

'Ex-president of Cuba Fidel Castro died in the early hours of the morning' was the headline that immediately greeted me.

As if on cue, the presenter turned to the news item that had caught my attention.

'Cuban state television announced that Fidel Castro, the former president of Cuba, died last night. The cause of death is not disclosed to the media. His brother, President Raul Castro, confirmed the news in a brief speech …'

There was a knock on the door. I realised that the door was still open. It was Salim with my cup of tea. He greeted me, but I barely acknowledged him, as my eyes and ears were still glued to the television, listening to every word being spoken.

Back home later that night, I had an early dinner and retired to my bedroom. I relaxed on my bed and picked up the book I had been reading. I removed the lovely bookmark with the image of a Sandpiper, opening to the page which I had been reading the previous night. As I stared at the page, my mind raced back to the time when I was a resident of Cuba, back in 1989. I could not believe that twenty-seven years had already passed. At that time, my husband was stationed in Havana for a couple of years as a guest of the Cuban government. Images of our lovely villa, with its foyer overlooking the garden, the beautiful Varadero Beach, the many diplomatic dinners that we had hosted, the couple of meetings with Papa Castro (as he was fondly called in Cuba), and Albert.

*Albert. Why did I suddenly remember Albert?* I thought to myself as the images of a handsome young man flashed in my mind, as if they were a part of my life just a few days ago.

Albert …

He was so different from my other clients. He was tall, almost six feet, but his slim frame made him seem taller. He had a pleasing personality and was always well groomed. What was striking about him were his deep eyes. I could see them staring at me.

The sound of the door opening brought me back to the present. It was my husband, Pankaj.

'Still awake?' he enquired.

'Just about to end the day,' I muttered as I kept the book aside and put off the reading lamp next to my bedside with the images of Cuba still occupying my thoughts.

There was water all around me. I could see very clearly for miles as the water merged with the sky. I felt like a fish swimming along with the beautiful marine life around me. Little fishes were talking to me, telling me their tales. I could touch the corals. I felt like a child playing with a new toy.

It was 1989. My first experience of scuba diving on my own. Pankaj and I had landed in Havana a month earlier. The initial days were spent in finding the 'perfect' house. Since then, with time at my disposal, I started exploring the island. I fell in love with Varadero Beach and the crystal-clear waters of the Caribbean Sea.

As I was lazing on the beach, the charming Diego lured me into taking a lesson in scuba diving, and I took to it just like a fish to water. I got my licence within a week, and here I was, all on my own. I did not want the hour to end, but the loud voice of Diego reminded me that it was time to go back to the real world.

I quickly changed and made my way to Cubalise, a diplomatic store where we did most of our grocery shopping. I had planned a dinner for a few of the Cuban ministers and some dignitaries the next day. This is a protocol I had to follow once every month during my stay in that country.

My maid, Benita, did our grocery shopping, but I wanted the dinner to be perfect in every sense and had decided to select the main ingredients. My maid had suggested a Cuban dish, *ropa vieja*, which is a lovely blend of shredded flank steak in tomato sauce, black beans, yellow rice, plantains, and fried yuca, with beer. I decided to add lobster and shrimp, which were my favourites. I made my way to the seafood section. There was a lot of variety on offer.

It was at this point that I saw him.

He was standing next to me, and I could see his reflection in the glass wall ahead of me. He had strikingly good looks, and I guessed he would definitely make heads turn when he walked into a room. After a moment, our eyes met the reflection of the other and paused. When realisation dawned, I quickly shifted my gaze and moved ahead. As I walked, I turned my head, and he was still there, probably still undecided on his selection.

I went ahead and picked up the other ingredients and made my way to the cash counter. As I passed the seafood aisle, my head turned almost involuntarily, and there he was, still standing by the seafood counter.

I was now intrigued for more reasons than one. He appeared to be an Indian. There were only a thousand Indians in Cuba. His appearance seemed so charming, almost like a movie star. Finally, seeing his almost stolid presence at the seafood counter, I decided to act. Walking up to him, I initiated a conversation.

'Hello, sir. May I help you?' I enquired politely.

He seemed a bit startled at the sudden sound of a voice which seemed to be directed at him. He turned around to face me with an enquiring look on his face.

'Ahh' was all he could mutter.

I suddenly sensed that my approach may have been too sudden, but I decided to continue, having already made the move.

'Hello, my name is Preeti,' I said with a wider smile. 'I was just enquiring if you need any help.'

He finally got hold of himself and reciprocated with a smile. 'Oh, hello. I am Albert.'

That was our first meeting. I helped Albert with his selection that day and also exchanged phone numbers.

The next day was busy. We were in a new country, and it took me a while to understand how the various services worked. Benita's husband, Carlos, came as a godsend. He connected me with the right people, and by the afternoon, the lawn was lit with bright lights; a row of tables had been arranged for laying out the food; a music system was in place with a local DJ who, rather reluctantly, agreed to play a selection of my favourite Beethoven tracks; and round tables and chairs were arranged randomly around the lawn, with a bunch of flowers to add a touch of elegance. It all seemed perfect.

The guests started arriving at 6 p.m. Pankaj and I were busy receiving them as they arrived and ushering them to the lawns.

'Hello, Mrs Pandit.'

I turned my gaze from the personal secretary of President Castro, with whom I was having a conversation.

I immediately recognised the short, portly gentleman who had addressed me. The voice belonged to Doctor Rehman Malik, a renowned neurosurgeon who practised at the Clinica Sistema Nervioso, reputed to be a very good hospital in Havana. We had met at a conference on mental disorders that I had attended during the last month. With his Indian parentage and reputation in the medical fraternity, I considered him an important person to be connected with during my stay in Cuba and accordingly had invited him to today's dinner.

I let Pankaj attend to the Personal Secretary while I went and greeted Dr Malik. 'Hello, Doctor. Glad you could come,' I responded warmly to his greeting.

'The pleasure is mine, Mrs Pandit,' he said with a slight bow and continued, 'You are looking lovely as always.'

I acknowledged the appreciation with a coy smile.

Doctor Malik continued, 'I need a small favour from you.'

A little surprised with the request but always wanting to help, I replied, 'Sure, Doctor. Let me know what you have in mind.'

'I have a guest with me,' he said as he pointed to his car. 'He was my last patient today, and as I finished, I suggested that he join me for this dinner.' Before I could respond, he continued, 'There is a reason that I want him to meet you and thought this may be a good occasion.'

I have always been very conscientious and believe in meticulous planning, which suggests that I am not a big fan of surprises. However, the second part of Dr Malik's request intrigued me. 'Sure, Doctor Malik. You can definitely ask your guest to join us.'

'That's so nice of you, Mrs Pandit,' the doctor said. 'This is not something I normally do, but something told me that you should meet him. I will go and get him.'

I waited at the gates and could see the doctor walk back to his car and speak a few words to his guest as he opened the front door.

Very soon, he and the guest were walking towards me. As they came nearer, I gasped in recognition of the person accompanying Dr Malik. The momentary break in his stride suggested that he too had recognised me.

'Hello, Albert.' I extended my hand towards him.

'Hello …' He thought for a moment. 'Preeti. I hope I got the name right?' he enquired.

'Oh, you two know each other,' said the doctor, interrupting our exchange.

'Not really.' Albert turned to the doctor. 'I happened to meet her at the supermarket the other day.'

'What a wonderful coincidence.' I smiled as I looked at the handsome face, which seemed more alert today compared to the rather confused demeanour he had exhibited the previous day.

I ushered them to the lawns and guided them to one of the tables.

I got busy with my other guests, and as the guests were having a drink after dinner, Dr Malik came up to me.

'Mrs Pandit,' he said, 'may I have a minute?'

In response to my nod, he continued, 'Would you be able to take some therapy sessions for Albert?'

Dr Malik seemed to be an expert at throwing surprises, and as he had a few hours earlier, he again left me searching for the right response. Sensing my state of mind, Dr Malik clarified, 'Albert has been visiting me for the past few weeks. He is under severe depression. I have prescribed medicines, but I feel he may be better served by therapy.'

My silence continued as my mind was trying to make sense of this new revelation.

After giving me a few moments to ponder, the doctor inquired, 'Well, what do you think?' and looked at me to elicit a response.

'I would be happy to offer therapy if it helps,' I said after quickly gathering my thoughts. 'However, I don't have a license to practise here.'

'Nothing to worry' was the quick reply. 'In Cuba, you need a licence only to prescribe medicines. Therapy is fine.'

I immediately posed my next question: 'Where would I have the sessions? I do not have an office, and I have never been in favour of having sessions at home.'

The doctor thought for a moment and said, 'You can use my office at the hospital. I don't use it when I am having surgeries.'

'No way, Doctor. That is not right,' the conscientious part of me responded.

The doctor was not about to give up in a hurry. 'You can have the first session there and see how it goes. You can then decide what to do next.'

'Are you sure, Doctor? Won't the hospital mind?' I asked.

'Well, not exactly as per the rules,' he countered with a smile. 'But if a few harmless indiscretions can help someone, then we can always bend some rules.'

The doctor seemed to have everything planned. Without even waiting for my response, he beckoned Albert to join us.

'Albert, I am leaving you under the good care of our dear lady here,' he said almost in a self-appreciatory mode.

'Oh,' Albert exclaimed, 'I did not know you are a therapist,' he said, ignoring the euphoria created by the doctor.

My thoughts were mixed. I was happy that an opportunity to pursue my passion was presenting itself but apprehensive about the way things were panning out.

Sensing that Albert was waiting for a response, I clarified, 'Well, I have been practising for many years now,' and I added, 'Would you want to meet me?'

'Dr Malik did mention that he was planning something very different for me,' he admitted with a tinge of excitement. 'I respect his opinion and will follow his recommendation.'

The assurance made me feel better about the situation. 'That's good, Albert. When do we start?'

He thought for a moment and responded, 'My calendar is not too busy on Tuesdays. I can always take a break around lunchtime if it suits you.'

'How about 2 p.m. on Tuesday?' I asked.

'Done.'

That was our second meeting.

The very next day, I called Dr Malik to know more about Albert. Albert was working as a senior vice president in one of the foreign banks which had set up shop in Cuba. He had been posted in Havana a year earlier. He was originally from Singapore, with roots back in India. This was a huge coincidence. What would be the odds of two people of Indian origin, who were residents of Singapore, now being on a business visit to Cuba? Destiny can indeed surprise you. Albert was living with his wife in a plush apartment a few blocks away from where I lived. Dr Malik was treating him for severe depression and had put him on a high dose of medication.

I waited for Tuesday with more than a tinge of anticipation.

The dinner had been well received by the dignitaries. Some of them even called up Pankaj and thanked him personally. I had begun to enjoy my stay in Cuba.

## 2

Tuesday arrived, and I reached Clinica Sistema Nervioso at 1 p.m. The hospital was a rather modest single-storeyed structure, surrounded by trees, which gave it the appearance of a hotel. I entered the building and made my way to the reception.

'*Hola, señora. Puedo ayudarlo.*' The lady at reception greeted me with a broad smile.

I had picked up a little Spanish over the last month, and these were the words which I probably heard more than any others. I made a mental note to prepare an appropriate response in Spanish. For now, I had to make do with my English.

'Good afternoon, *señora*. I want to meet Doctor Rehman Malik.'

'*Cita?*' (appointment), she asked.

'Personal visit,' I explained.

She picked up the intercom and spoke to someone.

'Up floor, office,' she replied in broken English while showing three fingers and pointing to the right with her hand. I guessed this was an indication for number 3 on the right.

With a polite show of gratitude, I headed to the stairs. The wall behind the reception was adorned with the names of the nineteen *especialidades* (specialities) that the hospital catered, which I thought was impressive for its perceived size. Even more impressive was the list of doctors, more than fifty of them, who were probably affiliated with the hospital. With an enhanced opinion about the stature of the hospital, I found my way to Dr Malik's office on the first floor. The third door on the right had the nameplate 'Doctor Rehman Malik (Neurologia)' affixed on it, so I did not have to rely on my guesswork anymore.

I knocked on the door and entered. His office was bright, with sunlight coming from the big window right across the room. On one side was a huge cabinet filled with books, while a table with chairs occupied the other side. The wall behind the table where Dr Malik was seated had several framed certificates with the name 'Doctor Rehman Malik' prominently displayed on them while the man himself was seated on a leather chair behind the wooden table. Lovely artefacts on the table were neatly arranged around a vase with fresh flowers, which gave an indication of Dr Malik's artistic tastes.

The little apprehension that the fastidious me had before coming here about the room not being suitable for therapy was laid to rest within those few seconds.

My visual survey was interrupted by Dr Malik's deep-throated voice. 'Hello, Mrs Pandit, please take a seat.'

'Thank you, Doctor,' I responded warmly and added, 'You do have a nice office here.'

'Glad you liked it. It will be your office for the next hour,' he said with a chuckle.

'That is your privilege, Doctor,' I said with respect. 'I am just using it for some time with your permission.'

Dr Malik got up from his chair and walked to the coat stand to pick up his coat. As he put it on, he beckoned me to take his chair, which I did reluctantly.

'I will inform the receptionist that you will be in my office doing some paperwork for me,' he said.

As he shut the door behind him, I surveyed the office once more. It looked even better from this chair.

I created a mental picture of how I would want the furniture arranged.

Accordingly, I moved the guest chair to the other end of the room and turned it to face the wall behind me. Someone sitting there could now directly see the sky through the big window. I ensured that there is a fair distance between the chair and the wall in front. I then moved the chair that I was sitting on from behind the table and positioned it such that I would be able see the person without any physical obstruction. I sat on my chair and visualised the scene. I covered the window with the curtains, allowing only a small opening right in front of the chair that Albert would sit on, for a little sunlight to come in. The perfectionist in me gave a thumbs up. It was now a matter of waiting for Albert.

The clock above the door showed 1:47 p.m.

Albert entered a few minutes before 2 p.m. I was immediately drawn to his striking features as well as his overall demeanour. He was dressed in a formal white shirt and black trousers, probably because he was coming from work, with a black jacket completing his professional look.

I beckoned him to sit on the chair, which I had so carefully arranged.

I offered him a glass of water from the jug kept on the table, but he politely refused.

In a soft tone, I said, 'Albert, be comfortable. I suggest that you relax for a few minutes.'

A few minutes silence followed, during which time his gaze was initially fixed on the ground, then towards me. As I looked into his deep eyes, I realised for the first time that they seemed to contain an ocean of sorrow and were waiting to pour their contents on an eager recipient.

He finally spoke in a hesitant voice. 'I was looking forward to this session.' He paused. He ran his fingers through his well-maintained mop of hair and shifted his gaze to the window in front of him.

I sat in silence while resting my hands on the armrest. As a therapist, I had learnt the value of silence as a wonderful tool to let the person go deep within and reach places where he had never gone or was afraid to go.

'I don't like to share my personal details with anybody,' he continued as he rolled his upper lip, looking for the right words. 'When I met you, I was initially blown away by your beauty and then by your very calm and soothing persona.'

Another important trait of a therapist is the ability to focus the discussion on the subject at hand.

'Tell me more about yourself?' I changed the subject.

He paused as he was required to change his train of thought.

'I don't know who I am and how I feel these days. I haven't genuinely smiled or felt joy at home for such a long time. I don't even know how that would feel.'

He sighed. I gave him the space to continue. He appeared nervous, almost tense. His gaze was on the floor as he was attempting to break through his own barriers and open up to someone.

'My life has been a hell right from my childhood. I have grown up watching the explosion of emotions when Mum would see Dad come home drunk. She would feel so helpless every time Dad would come home smelling of alcohol. Mum would either coldly stare at him or start shouting at him. That would lead to an argument, and she would talk about the past and how fate had been cruel to her. If she happened to be angry with my brother and me that day, she would say mean things to us.'

It was a genuine outpouring of his emotions.

'Due to these daily squabbles in the family, I started smoking at the age of 12 and drinking by the time I was 16. I also got into antisocial behaviour, like flirting with girls. I gravitated towards people I can always depend on. I gained pleasure in certain ways.'

I just nodded in acknowledgement and maintained a neutral expression.

He immediately clarified, 'I gave up smoking two years ago because it was affecting my health, and I drink occasionally, in social situations. I also got into many relationships, but none have been good. I get very intense in the beginning, but within the matter of a few weeks, I tend to lose feelings. Probably the process of getting to know the person is what attracts me the most,' he confided.

I made a note to delve into the relationships in one of the sessions. For now, I wanted to let him kill his own demons, and the first thing is always about bringing these demons out into the open from the dark corners of his mind, where they become parasites and influence his thoughts.

He continued slowly, almost halting after every word and searching for the next. 'I feel choice-less, even though I can see I have so much freedom. I find myself not doing things for my mum, my girlfriend, my dad, and my brother. Yet, I imagine in my thoughts all the actions I should or want to do for them.'

He seemed forlorn on that chair and so vulnerable. As a therapist, I had trained myself to control my emotions and always have an invisible veil between the client and myself.

His monologue continued. 'We are the best and the worst of our parents. In a restrictive home, we are always told that everyone is dangerous and we should not be friendly with others. We learn the habits of our parents. I fear that I am looking at everyone with suspicion. I felt the same kind of fear when my dad was angry with me, and I didn't want to approach him about it. I felt the same kind of fear and confusion that I imagined my brother must have felt when we were younger, and I was angry with him for looking at me in the mornings.'

His shoulders were stooped, head low. His face had despondency written all over it.

'How much responsibility should I take? How much do I have to pay? When can I stop feeling guilty? How can I provide a reprieve to my fear, anxiety, and guilt?'

Lots of questions which we needed answers to over the next few sessions.

I offered him a glass of water to wet his parched throat and to help him come out of the flood of negative emotions that he seemed to be drowning in. He drank the water and shifted in his chair.

He looked at me and started on a different track. 'There is this band that I have liked since long, but I lost touch over the last few years. Recently, I got an opportunity to connect with them again. I listened to their songs in a language I barely comprehend. Yet the stories, the music videos of the songs they sing, make me really appreciate what I have or want to have.'

There seemed no link between what he had been talking about earlier and his last revelation.

'I think about how one of their original singers—there were three—committed suicide. And now they have a new singer replacing him. I feel so angry inside. How could they replace him? I feel so sad he is no longer around. I hope they know the joy and gratefulness their band has brought to people who feel like I do when I listen to their songs.'

I finally interjected, 'Albert, what did you learn from this incident that you just narrated?'

He did not seem to hear me and continued, 'Death is so close to us. Nowadays, I imagine myself watching someone I love die. My girlfriend, I watch her coffin enter the fire at the crematorium, and I see myself standing there without any reaction. When I go to my room, I break down. Sometimes, I would imagine, during the "entering the fire" phase, that I would break down, and my brother would always be there. I would tell him I don't want people to console or touch me, and he would listen and follow my instructions. He would prevent people from coming near me. Then I would cry while placing my hand on the glass. It would shatter and burst into flames. I would float down to the coffin and lie with it as it entered the flames. No one would get hurt when it burst into flames. It would be like a sacred fire, warm and red.'

Albert was not in the room anymore. He was in a world where everyone seemed to be against him. In that world, people he loved were dying and leaving him all alone with his sorrows.

It was time to bring him into the real world. I was a little louder this time.

'Albert, how can you come out of this situation?'

He turned towards me and after a pause responded, 'For a long period in my life, though I can't recall when it started, I had begun hoping that something inspirational would occur to me, so that it could drive me towards something. It would make me ambitious. However, this has not occurred. Sometimes, I would go so far as to imagine perhaps if someone died or someone left me, maybe then I would get myself together and move. This thought would probably have come from watching too many "hopeful" movies, where the protagonist would always find themselves in the lowest points of their lives. Then suddenly something would occur, and they would pick themselves up and go.'

I seized the moment.

'Albert, let's talk about the movies that you mentioned. When the protagonists are in real trouble, you said something would occur. What is this something?'

His eyes were focussed on me as if waiting for me to continue.

'Albert, it is the protagonist's will, inner strength, and resilience which help him come out of the situation. It is only in fairy tales that a genie appears and grants you three wishes.'

I wanted to make him understand that he is responsible— not for the situation he finds himself in but for doing whatever is necessary to come out of the situation. That is the awareness which opens the mind to therapy.

I spoke to his ego and his sense of self-esteem. 'You are a highly respected professional and have a wonderful career ahead of you. Yes, your past has not been as good as it has been for many others, but history is full of people who have risen from the depths of misery to reach the heights of success, and the same history also tells us how they did it.

'Albert,' I enquired, 'do you have a habit of reading?'

'Yes, I do,' he replied.

'I want you to start reading the autobiographies of legends and get inspired by them. You don't create anything more or anything less than what you think in your head. You become what you are thinking. We need you to be in a highly inspired state of mind in all our sessions. Would you do that?'

'Yes, I will,' he accepted just as an obedient student would in response to a teacher's instructions.

'That's good. When do we meet again?' I asked.

'Are we done?' he asked with a sense of innocence which made him seem even more vulnerable.

I smiled. 'Yes, Albert. Done for today.'

'Can we meet on Saturday?' he enquired after some thought.

'Fine with me. Saturday, 2 p.m. is confirmed,' I replied.

I stood up and walked towards him. His face was still flushed with the variety of emotions that he had experienced, but there was the hint of a smile.

We bid our goodbyes. I sat for some more time in the room and gathered my thoughts.

Albert had a difficult past which was negatively influencing his present. I would need to help him detach.

The session with Albert was my first in the last three months due to my preoccupation with the Cuba relocation. As with every session, I felt a sense of satisfaction for doing something which I was probably born to do.

# 3

The week was very pleasant. The weather was warm and bright, just as I like it. I did a lot of reading, went for long walks on the lovely beaches of Varadero, and dabbled in some painting.

Albert came into my conscious thought on a few occasions, but I put them aside. I believed in maintaining a balance between my professional and personal life and had been successful so far.

Cuba was going through an economic crisis that year, and the overall mood of the capital city was sombre. However, that did not stop the steady flow of American and Spanish tourists from visiting the city. Although it is a sprawling metropolis, its old centre retains an interesting mix of Baroque and neoclassical monuments and a homogeneous ensemble of private houses with arcades, balconies, wrought-iron gates and internal courtyards. President Fidel Castro was almost revered by the majority irrespective of the economic issues. I understood from my conversations with locals that the president was a prime assassination target for many countries and groups.

On most days, I would hear my maid, Benita, call out to me from the courtyard, *'Señora ... señora, ven aca Papa Castro. Ven aca ver Papa Castro'* (Come here and see Papa Castro).

I would come out to see his cavalcade passing in front of our gates and catch a glimpse of his bearded frame sitting in the back seat. A few minutes later, another cavalcade would pass through and then another. I realised that these were decoy vehicles carrying someone with a resemblance to the president. I was looking forward to an opportunity to meet the leader in person.

I had not spoken to Pankaj about the session with Albert yet since he was very busy with his work. I consulted my acquaintances from the government about the chances of renting an office. I realised that I could not rent a space for any commercial activity due to my dependant status. With no option available, I spoke to Dr Malik and requested him for the use of his office space on Saturday. He gladly agreed.

I was in his office much before the scheduled appointment and on Dr Malik's exit, made the necessary changes to the furniture, and waited for Albert's arrival. I drew the curtains to avoid the glare of the sunlight.

He walked in on the stroke of the hour. He was dressed in casuals today. A yellow T-shirt tucked into his baggy pants and his brown sneakers did justice to his lean frame. The lovely fragrance of his perfume spread throughout the room.

'Good afternoon, Albert,' I greeted him as I extended my hand. 'How are you today?'

'Good afternoon, Preeti. I am very well, thank you,' he responded softly.

His hand felt cold and was limp.

I beckoned him to the chair.

'Preeti ... um ...' he started to say something and stopped.

'Go on, Albert,' I coaxed him.

With a lot of hesitation, he asked, 'Can you open the curtains please?'

'Sure, Albert,' I said and walked to the window. 'You like the sunshine just like me?'

He smiled nervously and said, 'It is too dark in here.'

I opened the curtains just enough for some light to come into the room.

'I am tired,' he said as soon as I had taken my seat. 'I have a headache.'

I did not react.

He continued, 'This week has been bad at home and in the office. I felt good after meeting you on Tuesday. Your calm presence and soothing voice made me feel relaxed.'

'That's good, Albert,' I said. 'We are here to get your life back on track. The more open you are, the faster we will be able to do that. Sit in a comfortable position and relax. There is no hurry,' I assured him.

I wished for a therapist chair.

He sat back and extended his leg to get into a more comfortable position. He rested his head on the high back of the chair and closed his eyes. He remained in this position for close to ten minutes, and I let him be.

'Albert, Albert,' I called out to him gently, 'are you OK?'

He opened his eyes with a start as if he had just come out of deep slumber. He regained his orientation and slowly moved into an upright position.

I repeated the question, 'Are you OK?'

'I am sorry,' he said with a tinge of embarrassment.

'Albert, when we are in a session, you decide what we need to do,' I explained to him. 'You decide what we need to talk about, when to start, and when to end. Please do not be sorry for anything that happens in the session. Let me assure you that we are here for you.'

'Thank you so much,' he replied with his hand on his heart. 'Let me tell you that your calm presence and soft voice really make me want to tell everything to you.'

'That's good, Albert.' I seized the moment to bring the session back on track. 'What would you like to talk about today?'

'My wife, Anna, didn't go to work earlier this week,' he said with a sudden show of anger, 'so I told her that this absence from work was not going to do good and she needed to be on the move.'

It was a rather abrupt start.

He continued, 'She snapped, "Don't bring me down. I'm a designer, and I know what I have to do."'

I listened intently.

His gaze was now down on the floor in front of him, almost staring at it, as if he was straining to recollect the events that he wanted to share.

He went on, 'My wife said, "My mother asked me to visit her next month in Singapore." I suggested, "My sister is getting married in the next two months, so it is better to combine your mother's trip with the wedding." My wife did not like that and started abusing me again. She left home on Wednesday and just returned last night. She was not even bothered about our children, who were with me.'

I noticed that he had again jumped from one incident to the other.

He continued, 'I am not able to concentrate on my work. I just aimlessly do my tasks. I am tired. I feel demotivated. I feel even bad when I know I can perform so much better without this stress.' He shifted nervously in his chair.

Sensing a pause in his narration, I asked, 'Albert, you talked about an incident with your wife. You also mentioned that this stress is affecting your performance at work. What is concerning you more?'

A therapist needs to ask questions which the other person had never felt a need to answer or whose answer he did not want to hear.

His eyes told me that he was pondering over my question. 'I am not able to think clearly. Right from the time I was about 16 years of age, I have been under stress due to all the family issues.'

I interjected, 'How would you describe the family issues?'

'Everyone had a problem with each other. There were days and months when we would not talk to each other. My family was stressed due to my brother. My mother was unhappy. She is an ambitious lady, but my father's family did not allow her to work. Father was a bit hard on her. On certain occasions, she wanted to kill herself ...'

I realised that Albert had the habit of shifting from one topic to another randomly. This was the appropriate time to focus his thoughts on one subject and delve deeper into it. Since his thoughts were on his mother, I thought it appropriate to let him stay there. 'Please tell me more about your mother,' I said.

His deep eyes looked in my direction before again settling down on the floor in front of him.

'My mother does not like me,' he murmured under his breath.

I waited patiently for him to continue, but he continued staring at the floor.

'What makes you think so, Albert?' I enquired.

'She does not like me or my brother, Alwin,' he muttered. 'She was always angry with us. Her rage would feel like lightning and thunder.' He cringed as he said this. 'It would come down hard, without any predictability. She would vent her anger on us for many hours, sometimes even for a week. Then the storm would pass for a day or two before she started again.' He looked at me now. 'It was tough to be a child in my house.' His face showed resentment.

'Why do you say that?' I asked.

He thought for a moment, probably trying to recollect an incident which would answer my question. 'Once, my mum restricted me from going to Australia on a school trip with my friends. Not everyone in my class got chosen to go, and I was so elated that I got chosen,' he said with a smile, probably the first time I saw it today. 'I remember my mum waking me up one night and sitting down with me along with my dad. It was dark. My mum explained that she felt it wasn't safe for me, so I couldn't go,' he recollected. 'I was crushed. I felt so sad and helpless that I couldn't go.'

He looked at me as if to say that he had proved his point.

'What made her angry?' I prodded.

'It could have been anything. Sometimes there was no reason. There would be showers of "bloody shit" and so much foul language that I cannot say to you.'

I could see a few tears welling in his eyes. Albert was in the moment.

'What specifically would make her angry?' I asked.

His downcast eyes suggested that he was searching for the right response. 'There was one New Year's Eve when I stayed out at a friend's house. This made my mum very uncomfortable. She even called up and threatened to inform the police if I did not come home immediately.'

Wanting to understand another dimension of the relationship with his mother, I said, 'Mothers are always concerned about their children. Wasn't this her way of showing concern?'

His retort was immediate and voice loud. 'You haven't lived with my mum. She is so condescending, always sarcastic, so mean and cruel to my brother and me.' He paused for a moment to catch his breath. 'When we tried to respond, she would challenge us to stare at her. Her eyes were so menacing,' he said as he gestured to his own eyes. 'We would just stand in our spot, cry and shout back at her, but she would not stop. When we would say something that hurt her, she would come angrily towards us and hit us,' he sobbed. 'She would hit us everywhere,' and then he paused, 'but she would not hit our faces.'

His breathing was slow and heavy now. His slumped frame suggested that he was reliving the memories of the events that he was just describing.

Not wanting him to dwell too much in those unpleasant memories, I intervened.

'When did these incidents stop?'

He turned towards me with a dazed look. 'The angry outbursts and beatings stopped only a few years ago. We had our own rooms then, so we would run into our rooms and learnt to ignore her. She would still be shouting outside, but we knew that she was powerless and her words could not puncture us anymore. We also had other women to turn to,' he said almost in a relieved tone.

'When my mum couldn't shed her anger with her fists, like her father did to her, she would shed it with words, tone, and style.'

That was an important revelation.

I leaned towards him and said, 'Albert, your mother seems to have endured this kind of behaviour from her father, which may have affected her. She may be genuinely concerned about you. What do you feel?'

He shook his head vigorously almost rubbishing my suggestion. 'Perhaps you may think my mum is concerned about me. You are right. She is but she doesn't know her concerns well enough.' His voice was very loud now. 'It is every parent's prerogative to be worried about their children. It is natural. But there has to be a balance.'

He paused and continued as if he was almost thinking aloud, 'I have come to realise that my mum was more concerned about how she would feel,' he was analysing the situation now. 'She was always worried and so consumed by her fears of not handling her worries that she would avoid the situation by restricting me. Maybe she wanted me to feel how her parents were also breathing down her neck after she got married. They would tell her, "What about us. What will happen when we fall sick and you are not here?" Probably that was her worry, because she would always say the same thing to us when she was angry while sarcastically mimicking my grandma's tone.'

He shook his head. 'Everything was about her,' he said with a sneer. 'Just because she did not like going to some places to eat, because she didn't like the food there or the lack of cleanliness or the simplicity of the place, she would not allow us to go there as well. I also remember how pathetic her excuses were if she did not want me to wash the dishes. She would say, "I can wash faster." If I happened to complain about something while cleaning the dishes, she would say, "See, I knew this would happen. Let me wash the dishes." Just trying to help and knowing I can't makes me feel so frustrated—that I have to be firm and almost angry before she lets me wash the dishes. It is as if she is trying to test my patience.'

He was letting out all the emotions that were bottled inside him. His mother seemed to be a key figure in his life, and he was frustrated that the relationship was so bitter.

He continued, 'In the recent past, I have realised how negative I am, but then I realised how negative my mum is. She is like lightning, very fast and destructive with her words. Anything that does not fit her terms can be twisted into some cynical situation, thus justifying why that situation is a bad one to her. My mum is very jumpy, and she can react to any kind of conversation that opens with a tone of seriousness with wide eyes, almost like she is bracing herself to be sad or worried. She worries excessively. In a lot of ways, her worry has held my brother and I back from many situations that were important to us.'

I looked at the clock. It was 3 p.m. I was sure that this could go on for another hour. I was about to take the session to a conclusion when I sensed a sudden change in Albert's body language. His hands were now clasped together tightly, eyes closed, frame leaning forward, and his breathing became heavy again. I waited.

'My mum ...'

He stopped, shaking his head, probably searching for the right words.

'Go ahead, Albert,' I prodded.

His eyes still on the floor, he whispered, 'My mum had many affairs.'

I suddenly felt the silence for the first time.

Albert was sobbing now. I let him be alone with his emotions.

Slowly, I could see him releasing his clasped hands and resting his back on the chair. He seemed relieved now that he had disclosed something which had been bothering him for so long. He continued, but with more control.

'She had affairs with many men. So did my father. But I don't care about him. I know she was doing this to hurt him. I even had arguments with some of the men, but I knew my anger was towards her ...' He trailed off. 'She should not have done this.'

The clock was now showing twelve minutes past three. I proceeded to conclude the session.

'Albert, thank you for sharing details of your life,' I said, 'especially your relationship with your mother. In your opinion, your mother did not like you. Before we end, tell me some nice things about her.'

Albert smiled. I was now making him think of the better moments of his life.

'My mother is very intelligent. She is a wonderful artist. Her paintings are very good.' His face seemed radiant as he was now recollecting the positive aspects of his mother.

'She would have become a great painter if she got the opportunity, but neither, her husband, nor his parents gave her the freedom,' he sighed.

'What else?' I enquired in an attempt to make him think more.

'She was OK when she was in a good mood. She would take care of me when I returned from school and feed me good food,' he recollected with the smile still intact.

I seized the opportunity and said, 'Albert, be with these pleasant thoughts until we meet again. There is always a silver lining around every dark cloud. Unfortunately, we only focus on the darkness.'

He responded with a smile as he got up from the chair.

'When do we meet again?' I asked.

He checked his pocket diary and replied, 'Let's meet on Tuesday. That's a relatively light day for me.'

'Same time?' I asked.

'Yes,' he replied. The smile brought a twinkle to his eyes. He looked even more handsome.

'I have a request,' he said hesitantly. 'Can we meet some other place? It is very suffocating here.'

'OK, Albert, we will meet some other place,' I promised.

'Albert, do you visit the beach often?' I asked.

'Well, sometimes,' he replied.

'I would like you to drive down to the Varadero Beach tomorrow early morning and just walk on your bare feet along the water's edge.'

He gave me a quizzical look. 'I don't like the crowd,' he said, and his face showed his dislike.

'Trust me, Albert. Just walk for an hour.'

'OK, Preeti,' he finally responded. 'Let's meet on Tuesday,' he said as he stood up.

'Yes,' I replied, 'I will give you a call on Monday and tell you where we will meet.'

I was sure that we needed a different setting for our next session.

## 4

I spent the Sunday scouting for a place where I could hold the next few sessions. My search led me to this wonderful lounge at Hotel Ambos Mundos, near Hemingway beach. This was a hotel where the famous author Ernest Hemingway stayed during his time in Cuba, hence the name of the beach. The hotel had an old-world charm and was tucked away in a silent corner of the rather busy part of the city. The lounge at the back of the hotel overlooked the sea and was generally deserted during the afternoons.

I had found my therapy room.

I called Albert on Monday and informed him about the new venue.

I reached Hotel Ambos Mundos by 1:30 p.m. and was happy to see just one person in the lounge. I chose a corner table from where the beach was all one could see. I would sit on the side facing the lounge, and Albert would be sitting facing the beach.

Having done the mental preparation, I sipped my coffee as I waited for Albert.

Like the previous sessions, Albert was punctual. He was in his business attire, and as I watched him walk in from the entrance to our table, he could be mistaken for a model strutting the ramp, except for his face, which was still brooding. I needed to work on that.

We exchanged pleasantries and made ourselves comfortable in our respective chairs. Again, the fragrance of his perfume filled the air.

I asked him, 'Would you like some coffee?'

He accepted the offer. 'It will help my headache,' he said, raising his eyebrows.

I noticed that he was very prone to headaches and made a note to speak with Dr Malik about it.

I started the session. 'We are meeting at a new place. I believe that a change of scenery brings out new thoughts. How are you feeling today?'

His deep eyes turned to the ocean behind me and became one with it.

'Hmmm …' he started to say something and stopped.

I looked into his eyes and encouraged him to continue.

'This place is so much better than the office. I felt suffocated there.' He cringed. That was the second time he was using the word to describe the office. 'I don't like to be in dark places. It seems to remind me of my own life. I want to break the shackles of darkness and embrace the warmth of light,' he confessed.

'Thanks for sharing that with me Albert,' I acknowledged. 'This is more to your comfort, isn't it?'

'Yes, Preeti.' He smiled. He was so genuine when he did that.

'How was the walk on the beach?' I asked, referring to my suggestion last week.

'Well …'

He again hesitated. I waited.

'It was crowded … I did not like it … I went back home,' he stammered.

'No problem, Albert. We will go there together next time,' I assured him softly.

That brought a smile to his face.

'I would love that,' he said. 'In fact, I feel so much better when I am with you. I don't share my personal details with anyone; I don't know why I feel like sharing everything with you,' he admitted.

The waiter brought the coffee. I acknowledged his comment with a nod and used the break in the conversation to get into the session.

'What would you like to talk about today?' I asked.

'I am confused,' he said after a moment's pause. 'There is so much going on in my life. I don't know where to start.'

Sensing his situation, I suggested, 'You spoke about your mother the other day. How was your relationship with your father?'

Albert was in a state of mind akin to an avalanche of thoughts and emotions running through it. He needed someone to channel his thoughts. The nod of his head and shift in his gaze suggested that he was now trying to focus on the subject.

'I did not see much of my father. He would work in the city,' he started.

'He was never around. He did not take an active part in our lives. Even our birthdays were celebrated as a favour to us.'

He was again getting into the zone, and I let him get there.

'I always feel that if he had paid more attention to the house, all of us would be doing much better today.'

'Would you have conversations with him?' I asked, trying to structure his thoughts.

'He would always be very quiet. He did not like us being childish and playful, but he would not say anything, just sit there quietly,' he recollected, and then, with a slight grin, he added, 'I would even indulge in antisocial behaviour to distract myself and get a reaction from him. Initially, he would shout but then would only look at me with anger and disappointment.'

He was in the moment now.

'I would have preferred if he had scolded me. At least, this way, he would have talked to me.'

An overindulgent mother and a nonexpressive father. Life wouldn't have been easy.

'How was his relationship with your mother?' I enquired, wanting some insights on all the three relationships.

He gave me a sarcastic smile, but his eyes conveyed sadness.

'The only relationship between my dad and mum was conflict. My mum would always threaten to divorce my dad. My dad would either be completely silent or go berserk with his loud shouting. Would you like to live in such a house?' he asked with a shake of his head.

I remained silent.

'My dad always felt that my mother should be doing everything: cooking, cleaning after her children, and so on. He was always controlled by his parents.'

'Was this a sign of a soft corner for his mother?' I wondered aloud.

'My dad tells me that when I was younger, he did not divorce my mum because she couldn't fend for herself, which may be true. At other times, he would tell me that he did not divorce her because of my brother and me.'

Albert looked at me and whispered as if afraid that someone might hear him, 'As I grew up, I began to realise he wasn't doing it because of himself.'

'Hmmm,' I muttered in response.

'My dad had a strange habit of reacting to everything with surprise; it almost feels like some of our decisions can be shocking to him.'

'OK.' I nodded, waiting for elaboration.

'The matter could be very mundane, but he would react with surprise. Like if my brother went for a run before lunch, he would react with a moment of surprise. His reactions can be overdone, making him jumpy at times. I would get irritated by this.'

He paused. I waited and then came in, 'Albert, did you love your dad?'

The response was quick. 'No. I did not really care about my dad's feelings or about how I felt for him. I only became aware of my annoyance at him after the first time I broke up with my girlfriend, when he asked me *that* intrusive question. Between my father and mother, I am more afraid of and angrier with my father. While I am angry with my mother and even afraid of her, she never threatened me with physical harm. My father's rage is the most intimidating. With my mum, sometimes I could shout back. Though it would be ineffective, at least I could get something out of my system. My father would be silent, but you could tell he was boiling inside. Most times, as I understood, he would come home from work in a drunken state and just explode at my mum. He would say mean things to her.'

Albert surely had a lot of sympathy for his mum, but there was another aspect which needed to be understood.

'Was your dad physical with you?' I asked, knowing this was an important aspect of any relationship.

'If I did something to piss him off, he would threaten me with a knife. If I was rude to him, he would say, 'Don't make papa kick you.''

I could see him cringing as he said this.

'Albert, it's OK to feel what you are feeling towards your dad,' I comforted him without being sympathetic. 'Can you share some of your good memories with him?'

'I don't care for my father' was the immediate retort. 'I wish I had a father who would keep his family happy, protected, and safe. He would understand what my mother and I were going through. He would care for his wife's feelings more and not be influenced by his family. Even though my father had extramarital affairs, I never bothered about them.'

The last comment showed complete disdain for his father.

I glanced at the clock. Almost 3 p.m.

'Have you spent time with your grandparents?' I asked since they had come into his narrative many times today.

'My parents decided to send me to Madras to stay with my grandparents after high school. The moment I moved there, they treated me like a guest. They did that because my father sent word to his father. I had to live with them. Grandmother would talk to me as if I was a burden on her. My grandfather was caring, but he would be influenced by my grandmother to say nasty things. But a lot of times, I empathised with how my mum lived in that house. I realised how my brother also lived in the house for one and a half years.' He was almost glowering now.

'I hate them,' he concluded.

I waited for Albert to continue.

'Would you like to share something more about your grandparents?' I asked.

He thought for a moment and replied, 'No. I hate them. I don't want to talk about them.'

Albert had this habit of getting so involved with every memory. It was as if he was squeezing the emotions of that moment and letting them override his present state of mind. It was, therefore, necessary to up his energy level every time he recounted an emotional episode from his past.

I needed to disassociate the memory of these bitter incidents with the emotions.

'Albert, your jacket looks so good on you,' I commented without appearing too coy.

That helped in getting him to the present.

'Thank you, Preeti,' he said with a sheepish grin. 'It's my favourite.'

'You do like to dress up well. I like your sartorial sense.' It was a genuine confession.

'That's so nice of you,' he said softly.

In this mood, his looks and his personality shone through.

*I am sure he has had a few girlfriends*, I thought. *That will be the topic of our next session.*

'Why don't you wait here and have a drink to rejoice the journey that you are on?' I suggested. He nodded in agreement.

'Let's meet on Saturday,' I said. 'This time in the morning, on the beach. How about 7 a.m.?'

There was no hesitation this time.

## 5

Cuba is a small island country but the largest of the Caribbean islands, with a population of around 6 million. The country is known for its beaches, often called the 'jewels of the country'. Its beaches are an attraction for tourists from all over the world. The best among the many beaches is Varadero Beach. The almost straight 25 km stretch of white sand runs across the entire peninsula and in combination with the blue and green crystal-clear waters of the Caribbean Sea, presents an enchanting view. The waters are so clear that you can spot a variety of marine life from the surface. Coral is abundant. These waters provide a perfect setting for wayfarers to indulge in some snorkelling and for the more adventurous to experience scuba diving.

The sky draping itself in a spectrum of vivid colours as the sun rises from the land behind us is a spectacle, and you cannot but wonder at the magic of nature. It was at this magical hour that I had asked Albert to join me. I was in my tracksuit and sneakers considering the time of the day and the location. The cool breeze blowing from the sea ruffled my hair as I alighted from the cab. I had specified a meeting point, which is where I headed. To my pleasant surprise, Albert was already there.

He was dressed in a track pant and a T-shirt. His hair was rather unkempt, and the unshaven look was a departure from the prim and proper person I had been meeting during the past couple of weeks.

'Good morning, Albert,' I greeted him when I was close.

'Good morning, Preeti,' he responded and extended his hand, which was again limp.

'A wonderful morning, isn't it?' I asked as I looked around and took in the atmosphere.

'Hmmm' was his rather cold response.

Albert did not seem to be in a good mood, and in this state, people cannot think clearly and may not be open to receiving anything. I first had to bring him to a more stable state of mind.

'Would you like to walk by the water's edge?' I asked and started walking towards the water, leading him to a favourable response.

'Sure' was his monosyllabic answer.

'We have been meeting each other for about two weeks now,' I said. 'In these two weeks, you have shared a lot about your past. You have been very open and shown an urge to move your life onto a different plane. How is the Albert of today different from the Albert that I met two weeks ago?'

We were slowly walking along the water, and the sound of the waves filled the silence. There were just a few people at the beach, most of them jogging on the sands, so we had the beach almost to ourselves.

After what seemed an eternity, Albert spoke. 'Preeti, I have never been an outgoing person. I have very few friends, and my social circle is limited. Even with them, my interactions are ...' He searched for the right word and came up with 'measured'.

He continued, 'I don't know why, but since the time I met you and you spoke to me, I have been enchanted by you. Your lovely face, soothing voice, and pleasing personality made me feel so comfortable that I just opened my heart to you. Even I did not realise that there was so much inside me. It just kept coming out.'

We kept walking as he again retreated into this shell. I kept silent since I did not want to be a filler in his string of thoughts. My experience suggests that people who are introverts like to remain in their comfort zone by wearing the mask of a good listener. Rather than actually listening, they are just enjoying the comfort of not speaking. They add a few words to a conversation and then happily allow the other person to take over. As a therapist, my objective is to bring people out of their comfort zone. It is in the volatile and uncertain bends of our lives that real transformation occurs. Albert was the same. I waited.

He suddenly stopped and turned towards me. 'Please, help me,' he almost pleaded. 'I have had enough of this horrible life. My wife fought with me the entire night, and I have hardly slept.' The explained his appearance.

He continued, 'I have very bad dreams every night, and these memories keep coming back to me. I don't know how to come out of it. You are the first person I have met who I feel can really help me. I want to live a happy life where I have peace of mind.'

I started walking again, and he followed.

'Albert, the first step to the life you want to lead is to let go of your past,' I explained slowly, making sure that he was with me. 'To make that happen, we need to identify those disturbing memories and confine them to a corner of the mind where they don't bother us anymore. I want you to look at all these memories and pour them out. You have shared a lot about your relationships with your mother, father, and grandparents. I would like to know more about your girlfriends. Can we talk about them today?'

He seemed to feel assured with my response, as I finally saw a smile on his sullen face.

'Yes, I can do that,' he said.

We kept walking.

'I was having a horrible time at home, so I would find comfort in the company of girls. During my school days, I had flings with many girls. I don't remember having any feelings for them. I was only interested in the physical part of the relationship, and it gave me some relief from the constant bickering at home.'

'Did you have any serious relationships?' I asked.

He said, 'I had a girlfriend when I was in my college. Her name was Sangeeta. She was a very confident person. Once she would set up her mind on something, she would do it, whether other people liked it or not. When I was initially acquainted with her, I liked this trait, but later, I started to feel irritated. I didn't say it, but this is something which kept bothering me.

'Can you please elaborate on this feeling of irritation?' I enquired.

He stared at the sand in front of him and verbalised his thoughts as he had always done during our earlier meetings.

'I remember that she had once taken a holiday from school. I suggested that we should go to movies the next day. The next day, I felt lazy and asked her if we could go some other time. She was fine with it. Later in the day, I felt guilty about it and suggested we go for a movie in the evening. She refused, stating that I might only be doing it to fulfil my promise and not because I really wanted to. She also stated, "It's OK. I am fine if we don't go, because if I really wanted to, I would have gone anyway, regardless of anything." I could not stand it when she would just dismiss me like this.'

I waited a few moments and then urged him to continue.

'She was very possessive about everything, and during the early days of our relationship, I would throw away everything just to be with her. I now feel that I should have had more confidence in telling her what I wanted rather than only satisfying her. I would not be in the situation I am in. I feel contempt for her now,' he said, shaking his head and clenching his fists. 'I still remember an incident when my friend had asked me to travel with him on a trip. I was all excited and said yes but then realised that Sangeetha would ask me, "What about me?" and I said no to him.'

'You could have taken her with you,' I said, wanting to see if he had considered this option.

His retort was immediate. 'She had school at that time.' He quickly continued, 'I felt so guilty about leaving her behind. I was only thinking of her feelings and not mine. I remember feeling upset and helpless about it.'

I waited for a moment and then intervened, 'Please go on, Albert.'

He was searching for the right memories to come forth.

After a pause, he continued, 'I believe that the fault is with me. I would be initially happy in every relationship, but soon I would lose interest due to the responsibility it would bring.

'How about your wife?' I enquired, trying to steer his thoughts in a different direction.

A sarcastic grin appeared on his handsome face. 'My wife is the same. She wants everything to happen her way but will not say it. When I don't do what she is expecting, she gets cross and starts ignoring me.'

'Tell me more about her,' I said.

'Her name is Anna. It's been four years since we are married. She is a fashion designer and has her own business in Singapore. She had to leave her business and come with me to Cuba. She has always been independent, and it was a surprise that she even decided to relocate with me. However, immediately after coming here, she became very frustrated and threatened to go back home with our kids. With great difficulty, I managed to get her connected with a local design house, and they agreed to take her on contract. I had to make it look like an offer had come from them, or else her self-esteem would not have accepted it. Within a few days, she started complaining that the work here is so uninteresting. She would not go to work on many days, and when I try to reason with her, she just leaves the house and goes and stays in a hotel for many days. She does not care for our kids.'

In his entire tirade of about ten minutes, he did not say one positive word about her. This was probably another of his failed relationships. No wonder the guy was on medication.

We had probably walked a few kilometres before I realised that the sun was now visible over the many buildings that made up downtown Havana. My watch showed 9 a.m.

I stopped and turned towards him. 'Albert, you have shared many details about your life and the many relationships you have been in. You shared several bitter memories, which is a good thing, because now you can work on making them irrelevant in your present life. I would like to suggest something. Would you want to hear it?'

'Most definitely,' he said eagerly, 'especially coming from you.'

I ignored the last bit and continued, 'I understand that Saturday night is a wild night at Varadero Beach. There are many dance parties which extend well into the night. I want you to join one of these parties tonight. I want you to just let go.'

My suggestion got him off guard.

'No way,' he retorted. 'I don't like crowds, and I don't like parties.'

'Well, that's exactly why I want you to come here tonight,' I quipped, and I added, 'Get your wife along if you can find a babysitter.'

'She will not allow me to come,' he said with a cynical laugh.

'Albert, it was just today morning that you asked me to help,' I reminded him. 'I promised you I will, and I never said it would be easy. You have to do this for me.' That was inadvertent.

'OK, if you insist,' he said hesitantly. 'I will try speaking to her.'

We left for our respective homes.

## 6

We had a few more sessions over the next two weeks. Albert spoke more about his relationships, his dreams and his fears. He had a phobia for darkness, closed spaces, crowds and water. He never visited the Varadero Beach at night and join a dance party. He did, however, start reading the autobiography of Abraham Lincoln and shared some of the passages which had inspired him during our sessions. He also started visiting the beach every morning for a walk.

During these four weeks, we had sessions at the beach, the hotel lounge, and even a café outside his bank. During every session, Albert would pour his heart out and I would be the empathetic receiver. I would leave him with some thoughts and some actions and encourage him to reflect on the same. By the last week, he seemed more in the present. He would come to the sessions with a smile, and his handshakes became firmer. After every session, he would look at me with his deep eyes perched on his striking face, initially with a sense of gratitude but later with a growing sense of infatuation. I had been enamoured by his personality but had always maintained my professional distance and consciously never encouraged his subtle advances. On his part, Albert never crossed the line.

It was 10 a.m. on a Saturday. Eight weeks had passed since my sessions with Albert started. I had planned something very different today. Accordingly, I was waiting for Albert at the Varadero Beach Activity Center.

He arrived on time, as he had always done during the past four weeks. He had been an extremely disciplined student if I could call myself a teacher.

As we had agreed, he was in knee-high Bermuda pants and a loose shirt. His Ray-Ban glares accentuated his looks. He was definitely making a few heads turn as he walked towards me, looking so much refreshed as compared to the first time I had seen him.

'Are we ready to do something different today?' I asked after the initial exchange of pleasantries.

'What would that be?' he enquired with a tinge of nervousness creeping into his voice.

'You will soon see,' I responded and headed inside the activity centre. 'Follow me.'

I headed to the registration desk and spoke to the guy at the counter. Albert followed me with a quizzical look.

Once I had finished my conversation, I turned to Albert and said, 'Albert, your snorkelling lessons start today.'

'What?' Albert gasped. 'No way. Absolutely not.' He backed off and turned towards the exit.

I called out to him in an assertive tone, 'Albert, please come here. You don't have a choice.'

'I can't get into the water. I have told you I am scared to death when I am anywhere near water. The closest I have been to water is when I walk on the beach.' He shook his head vigorously. 'No way.'

I stood my ground. 'Albert, please listen to me. Either you are enrolling for this course, or this will be our last meeting. You decide.'

It was my turn to walk towards the exit. He came running behind me and made me stop near the exit. He was almost in tears now. 'I can't do this, Preeti. Please, I beg of you.'

I softened my tone. 'Albert, you have been living with many fears for thirty-two years of your life. Wouldn't you like to live the rest of your life as a free man who is not bound by his own fears, most of which have been created by circumstances? Your life has been adversely influenced by others, and it is time you break free from the shackles that bind you and bring forth the real you.'

He calmed down slowly, and his stiff body became more relaxed.

Seeing no escape route, he reluctantly agreed, 'Fine. I will do it for you.'

'Not for me, Albert. You are doing this for you,' I replied with a smile.

That was the beginning of a five-day course on snorkelling. The instructors were experienced enough to deal with clients like Albert who had never even dipped their head underwater.

I was using water therapy to release him from his fears. In a week's time, Albert was snorkelling off the coast on his own. I would join him on some of his trips and then have a conversation with him at the lounge. I could slowly see the transformation happening. He would smile more than before, and his thoughts were less about the past and more about what he would want to be doing. He would talk about his little children more and show me their pictures. Of course, he continued to have his episodes with his wife and mother, which would disturb him for a few days, but the change was visible.

I realised that now was the time for the next master stroke.

'What?' Albert said with an exasperated response.

We were sitting in the lounge on a Saturday afternoon after a snorkelling trip. Over a cup of coffee, I had stated, 'Albert, you could be cutting down your medication by half, and with immediate effect.'

'Are you sure?' he stammered. 'I mean ... I have felt tremors when I have delayed taking my medication by thirty minutes. How can I do this?'

'That's exactly the point, Albert.' I said calmly. 'You have been under the influence of people and have been too dependent on medicines to keep you going. I want to free you from that as well.'

'What about Dr Malik?' he asked.

'I have already spoken to him,' I assured him. 'However, it all depends on you and your mindset. Tell yourself that you don't need these medicines, and you can live without them. Do this with a positive frame of mind. In the fight between the mind and body, it is the mind which will always prevail.'

I had made this calculated move in consultation with Dr Malik. I knew this could backfire and take Albert back by a few months. However, I also knew that this was the only way he would be able to restore his life or rather live life on his own terms.

'Call me tomorrow afternoon,' I told him before we parted.

## 7

My phone rang at 4 p.m. on Sunday.

I answered it to hear the excited voice of Albert.

'I have done it,' he screamed. 'I can't believe it. I have not taken any medicines since morning, and I am fine.'

'That's wonderful Albert,' I responded with equal excitement, 'Are you feeling any discomfort at all?' I asked.

'None at all,' he answered. 'In fact, I am about to go for a drive.'

'That's good, but don't have any beers,' I cautioned. 'Let's celebrate one step at a time.'

'Sure, Preeti. Whatever you say.'

This was a major step in his journey, and he had passed with flying colours. One last step remained, and if he managed to clear that, I was sure that Albert would be free in every sense.

Scuba diving.

As expected, there was the initial pushback, and I had to use my powers of persuasion to again provide him with no option.

After two weeks of training, he was ready to try his first dive in the deep sea. We were in the boat which would take us a little off the coast. Our instructor, Diego, was with us. We were in our scuba-diving gear. I had experienced a few dives with Diego before, but this was Albert's first dive in the deep sea.

I could see his nervousness as his feet were continuously shaking. His hands were cold as they held mine tightly. Albert had not spoken since the time we sat in the boat, and I let him be.

'*Tiempo para saltar*' (Ready to jump), Diego said as the boat slowly came to a halt a few kilometres into the Caribbean Sea. The weather was lovely, just warm enough for the marine life to be closer to the surface. Under the clear blue sky, the expanse of water looked pristine and inviting.

We sat on the edge of the boat with our backs to the sea. With a shove, Diego pushed Albert into the water and after a few seconds followed him. I dived in after a few minutes. I was immediately transported to another world. I oriented myself and looked around to see Diego and Albert a few feet away to my right. I swam towards them and came next to Albert. I showed a thumbs-up sign. He responded by making the sign with both hands.

The therapy was over.

In the middle of the ocean, away from the world that human beings inhabit, Albert had found himself. He had undergone many weeks of struggle where he had to repeatedly come out of his comfort zone, and through his discipline, he had finally conquered his deepest fears. The goal was achieved. Some formalities needed to be completed.

My thoughts were broken by a tug to my arm. Albert was pulling me in the direction where Diego was heading. We followed him, and soon enough, we witnessed one of the most spectacular views one can ever see on this planet. We were amongst the coral reefs. Marine life of all colours, shapes, and sizes swam around us. The almost endless coral reefs at the bottom looked like a forest, with the trees fluttering in the breeze. Diego beckoned us to follow him to the top of a reef. He slowly picked up a piece of coral and handed it to Albert. I picked up one and marvelled at this wonder of nature.

I was all alone with my thoughts there. For the hour, we were underwater. I was not a therapist but a curious child wanting to capture every moment of this spectacular treat that was on offer. It required Diego to signal a few times before I came out of my spell and began my swim back to the boat.

Back at the activity centre, I took a quick shower and came to the waiting area to meet Albert. As soon as he saw me, he came forward and gave me a hug. On a couple of occasions in the past, he had attempted it, but I had consciously ignored them. This time, I was caught unawares, but I let it be. We remained in that position for some time before I stepped back. Albert held both my hands and looked into my eyes.

'You are my angel,' he said softly. 'I have never felt anything like this before.'

'Albert, I am flattered by all the nice things you have been saying about me right from the time we met about six months ago. You are a very attractive man, and any women would be attracted to you. I would count myself as one as well. However, I stand by my professional ethics and my moral values. You will always be a dear friend.' I released my hands from his grip.

We met one more time as a therapist and client at the hotel lounge. I had already spoken to Dr Malik and on his advice told Albert to stop his medicines completely. I was confident that this was a mere formality, and that's how it turned to be.

Albert moved on with his life. He divorced his wife and found a lovely Spanish girlfriend who turned out to be a lovely mother to his kids. He visited our home a few times as a family friend during our stay in Cuba. I never divulged his identify to Pankaj, and so it remains to this day.

## 8

Nature versus nurture is a debate that has been raging amongst scientists for a long time. From the initial sessions, I realised that his family was an integral factor of Albert's identity. Even though his issue was about his current relationship with his wife and his work, I recognised that wasn't the root cause of his problems. It was his upbringing and certain incidents in his past that were creating dysfunction in his life currently.

Let's put ourselves in the shoes of a 4-year-old child, who has a mother he is very attached to and a father who is not at all emotionally involved in his life. His memories of his father revolved around anger, frustration, and incompleteness. Albert grew up in an environment where he had seen his mother stifle her own ambition because his father and his mother's family did not allow her to progress. He had grown up learning that his father was only there as a trophy father.

At a very young age, Albert was sent away to his paternal grandparents' house. He had to uproot his life and move from Singapore to India, where he soon realised that he wasn't very welcome. While his grandfather was welcoming, his grandmother was not. He felt like an outsider in his own house. This is when he first realised the hurdles his mother and brother faced when they were living with his father's side of the family.

In Singapore, he developed a smoking habit at the age of 12 and started drinking at the age of 16. However, the greatest effect from his dysfunctional family dynamic was the way he viewed his love relationships. When he met me for the first time, he was married and had children. However, he had ex-girlfriends who he seems very attached to him even now. His nature had become moody and possessive.

When he was growing up, he had seen both his parents have extramarital relationships. While his father was abroad for work, his mother would see other men. He also had a few altercations with these men. This behaviour of his mother affected him deeply. He felt that he had always been shielded by his mother from any confrontations, so when he saw his mother with someone else, it was a breach of trust. Even when he gave his mother the ultimatum, it did not work. This loss of control was also something that shaped his worldview today.

Only after the basic physiological and safety needs are met can a person actually have a strong foundation to start building mental health, and only when the psychological needs of love and esteem are met can the person aim to achieve one's full potential.

In the case of Albert, even though his physiological needs were consistently met, since his youth, he had had his childhood home snatched away from him. He had to move in with his grandparents in a completely new country, which itself can be a traumatic memory. This may have caused his safety needs to be stifled.

Having a suicidal mother and an absent father surely was also a hit on his psychological needs. He did not have the consistency and security; a well-functioning family should provide. Furthermore, his clinginess to his mother and disregard for his father indicated that his esteem needs weren't being met either.

Albert has been having emotional and societal problems because, while growing up, his hierarchy of needs weren't met due to his dysfunctional family. This plus the traumatic incidents in his life had caused him to suffer depression, anxiety, and emotional dysregulation.

The human mind is gentle, and in one's formative years, it needs to be handled with care. However, the human mind is also resilient. With more dysfunction, it adapts to survive, to grow, and to nurture. Albert is a clear example of such a case.

Yes, he is moody, he is possessive, and he is having trouble. However, he is also a functional member of society. He believes in maintaining positive relationships. He gives his trust to his friends. He came into therapy and opened himself up to scrutiny because he cared—maybe more than he would like to admit.

And it's this care that is a hope for humanity. This is what separates us from the animal kingdom, and it is this care that pushes humankind to strive to do better for the future generation.

# CHAPTER 2

# THE TWIN SOUL

## 1

In the last thirty years, I have had the opportunity to touch so many lives in different parts of the world. During this wonderful journey, I have met many people who were struggling to cope with the vagaries of life and were seeking a solution. Every person was different, and every interaction has been a learning experience. Among all these interactions, there is one which has to find a mention here. Without a shadow of a doubt, it has been the most intriguing and definitely the scariest. I still get goose bumps when I think of it.

The universe works in mysterious ways. There have been times when the place where I was, and the time when I was there happened to be the right place and the right time. If I hadn't, on a whim, decided to enter a coffee shop on that particular day and time, I may never have met Sujatha.

That meeting changed my life, and those of a few others, in more ways than one.

It was one of those hot and humid days in Singapore. After my lunch, I had some spare time before my next session at 4 p.m. I was walking along the orchard road, browsing the new summer collection in the market. I had been window shopping for more than an hour, and the relentless summer heat made me crave for something cold to soothe my parched throat. I decided to treat myself to one of those premium cold coffees, which would help my body cope with the heat and also provide me with the extra caffeine to continue with the long and busy day ahead.

I was relieved to enter the cool environs of the Coffee Bean and Tea Leaf. I found a place in the far corner from where I could get a good view of the place. After all, watching people and their behaviour was a favourite pastime of mine. I took a few deep breaths before I proceeded to the counter and ordered a tall caramel macchiato.

The first sip of the lovely chilled brew rejuvenated me, and all my senses became extra receptive as I surveyed the place. Since it was a weekday, the place was sparsely populated. There were a few men in their business suits having an animated conversation. A few youngsters were working on their respective laptops. A girl in the far corner seemed to be in her own world, engrossed in the pages of a book. In a few minutes, the men left, and the coffee shop turned silent. It was in this moment of calm that I noticed her. She was sitting at the table just ahead of me. Probably it was her nervous demeanour that made me notice her, as she kept flicking her mobile phone and shaking her head. This caught my attention. She would get into deep thought for a few moments and then go back to fiddling with her phone. She kept moving her legs, showing signs of stress or nervousness. Even from where I was sitting, I could see the creases on her forehead. She was wearing a *churidar kurta*, a typical Indian dress, and her pleated hair was rather dishevelled. She was wearing a *bindi* on her forehead, which gave away her Indian origins. She must have been in her late forties. Everything about her suggested a person in some sort of anxiety.

Just as I was in the process of dissecting her, she burst into tears. The silence in the café was suddenly shattered, and the few guests looked up from whatever they were doing. I still don't know why, but I got up and walked up to her table.

'Hello, ma'am,' I greeted her softly.

She looked up, startled, possibly by the sudden intrusion into her space.

'Are you OK?' I enquired gently while keeping my distance.

She was sniffling now, and her tears had already consumed a handful of tissues. Seeing me volunteer, the others in the café got back to what they were doing earlier.

Her head still buried under a few tissues, she nodded.

'I am sorry for intruding your privacy. I was observing you for some time now, and I realised that something was bothering you,' I said in a gentle voice. 'My name is Preeti, and I am a psychotherapist.'

I just let the words linger.

She finally looked up. The tears had made a mess of her face, and her hair was all over the place.

'Do you need any help?' I asked softly.

'No, I'm OK,' she whispered, using a few more tissues to absorb the tears.

I waited for a brief moment and felt a genuine concern for the lady. I could not, however, insist that she accept my offer of help.

'This is my card. Do call me if you need to talk to somebody,' I said as I removed a card from my purse and put it on the table.

She glanced at it and murmured, 'OK.'

I returned to my table and finished my coffee. The lady seemed to slowly regain control of herself as I left the coffee house to continue with my day.

Many days passed, and the coffee house incident had become a distant memory.

A few days later, I was going through some case papers in my office when my phone rang.

I picked up the phone to hear a lady's voice.

'Am I speaking to Dr Preeti?' the voice asked.

From my experience, I could make out the accent to be distinctly South Indian.

'Speaking!' I replied

'Ma'am, my name is Sujatha … Sujatha Nair,' she said, stressing the 'H'. 'If you remember, we were at the coffee house a few days ago, and you gave me your card.'

I could not place her and tried to buy time with a pause.

'ma'am, I-I … I was not feeling too well that day and couldn't control my tears,' she said, trying to help me. 'You came to help me, and—'

'Oh, yes, I remember now,' I interrupted as the visuals of the coffee house scene began playing in my head.

'Can I meet you?' she inquired.

'Sure, you can,' I answered. 'You will have to come to my clinic.'

'OK,' she replied.

'When would you like to come?'

'I-I don't know,' she stuttered. 'You tell me.'

I quickly checked my appointments and spoke on the phone again. 'Can you come on Friday at 11 a.m.?' I asked.

She was quick to respond. 'Yes, yes, I will come.'

I took out my diary and pencilled in the appointment under the name of Sujatha Nair. Something was telling me that this case was going to be different—very different

## 2

Friday arrived, and I was in my clinic at 10 a.m.

I did my breathing exercises and settled down with a book.

Just past the hour, there was a knock on the door of my therapy room, and she entered. I placed the bookmark in the page I was reading and closed the book. I looked up and saw her enter. She was dressed in typical Indian attire, which seemed ill-fitting for her rather overweight frame. Her curly hair was oiled and neatly combed back. She seemed more composed today.

'Hello, Sujatha.' I stood up to receive her.

She took some measured steps and accepted my handshake. Her hands were cold.

I sat down and gestured for her to be seated in the chair on the other side of the table. She did so and remained silent. I waited for a moment and then initiated the conversation.

'Tell me, what brings you here?'

'I need some help for my daughter,' she responded.

Her voice was soft, and her narration was slow.

'What about your daughter?' I asked.

'She is not well, and I don't know what to do,' she replied. 'You came forward to help me that day. Probably, God has sent you.'

I could see the tears making their appearance. She seemed like a woman who had lost hope but had perhaps found a sliver.

'Sujatha, I have been practising therapy for close to thirty years,' I assured her. 'Please tell me about your daughter, and I will try to help.'

Her gaze was on the table separating us. She remained silent.

'Can I bring her to you?' she blurted out suddenly.

'Sure you can, Sujatha!' I continued calmly, 'But tell me something about her so I can be prepared.'

'She was a bright girl, but probably someone has cursed her,' she said under her breath.

'What's her name?' I asked without acknowledging her statement.

'Latha,' she said.

'How old is she?'

'Nineteen' was her monotone response.

I had to make her talk.

'Tell me about Latha,' I said and leaned back on my chair as if to give her some space.

'I am sure someone has cast a spell on her,' she continued from where she had paused earlier. 'She was always good in her studies. She was good at music. Why does she have to suffer?'

I believe everything that the other person says or does has some significance. Sujatha's responses, however, were not helping me understand what Latha's problem was.

I had to take her into confidence.

'I will try my best to reduce her suffering, Sujatha!' I said softly. 'But I cannot do that without your help. Both of us need to trust each other. I believe that you only want good to happen to Latha. So do I. Do you trust me?'

'Yes, I do, ma'am,' she said with a genuineness that gave me a lot of assurance.

'Thanks, Sujatha. Since you trust me, you need to tell me everything about Latha so that we can help her. Will you do that?' I enquired, trying not to sound too forceful.

That helped, and she started her narration.

For the next fifteen minutes, she spoke, and I listened. Her daughter had been unwell for close to a year now. She was not sure about the real problem, as she had heard multiple versions from different people whom she had approached for treatment. During the past year, she had knocked on the doors of psychiatrists and mental institutes but to no avail. She was confused and completely lost. She seemed emotionally and physically drained out. I would not gain anything by probing her more in this condition.

'Sujatha, you wanted me to meet your daughter,' I said.

'Yes, ma'am,' she answered quickly, and her body language suggested that was the only thing she had come here for.

'How about Tuesday at 11 a.m.?'

She agreed.

## 3

I had a wonderful weekend with the family. My daughter was visiting from abroad, and the entire family went for a short trip to Pulau Ubin. This is an island off eastern Singapore, and a stroll through Ubin takes one back to Singapore in the 1960s, with the simpler pleasures of life. We went for some shopping on Sunday. Monday was a relaxing day at home, as I had not taken any appointments. Come Tuesday, I was all refreshed.

The mother and daughter arrived at 11 a.m.

The daughter was as tall as her mother, but she was very thin and pale. Her hair was unkempt, and her skirt and top were not coordinated. Sujatha led her by hand as they sat down in front of me.

'Hello, Sujatha,' I greeted her.

'Hello, ma'am,' she said nervously. 'She is—'

'I asked you to take me to the lawyer,' the rather coarse voice interrupted Sujatha's introduction. 'Why have you brought me here?'

She was breathing heavily. Her fists were clenched, and her face was all red.

Sujatha held her hand and said softly, 'Beta, this lady will help you get better.'

'Amma, I don't want to meet this stupid lady,' she bellowed. 'I want to meet a lawyer.' She stomped the floor with her foot as she said that.

Sujatha was nervous now and looking at me for some help in dealing with the situation.

'Latha, I will help you with whatever you want,' I said gently. 'Tell me about it.'

She turned her gaze towards me. Her eyes were piercing, and if looks could kill, she would have murdered me.

'I don't want to talk to you,' she shouted so loudly that I was taken aback for a moment.

'Latha, that's OK,' I said, trying to remain calm. 'You don't have to talk to me if you don't want to. Why do you want to meet a lawyer?'

'I don't want to speak to you. Can't you understand, stupid lady?' Her voice was menacing. Her eyes were glaring at me, and they were filled with rage. Her entire body was shaking.

The pale-yellow light in the room was casting a shadow on her face. That, combined with her glowering eyes and coarse voice, made the setting very eerie. I had to think of an alternative approach.

I turned my attention to Sujatha. 'You were telling me that Latha needs a lawyer. Well, I have a friend who is a lawyer. I met him yesterday, and he is ready to help. He was asking me for more details. What should I tell him?'

I was hoping for a different reaction from Latha, but there was none. I persisted.

'Sujatha, you were telling me how Latha was good in her studies and that you were proud of her.'

Sujatha got the cue. 'Yes, she is really good in her studies. Right from her kindergarten, she would always be the best student in her class just like her sister Mala. She is very intelligent. She always tells us that she will become a doctor when she grew up.'

I glanced at Latha from the corner of my eye. She had moved her gaze to her mother now. As her mother said all the nice things about her, it seemed to calm her down.

'Oh, that's wonderful,' I applauded. 'She was good at music too?'

'She was initially not interested in music, but her sister, Mala, was very good …'

As Sujatha was talking, I was not only listening to what she was saying but was also watching Latha's body language. It's said that our bodies say so much more than the words we speak. Although Latha did not speak much, I heard her.

I had received some clues, but I would need some time to go through my mental notes.

'Let's do one thing,' I interjected. 'I will get my lawyer friend to meet us here on Friday. Sujatha, can you come with Latha and meet him?'

Sujatha gave me a quizzical look. I realised this was not going to be easy. Latha continued with a slightly toned-down expression of anger.

I got up and led them to the door. My attempt to shake Latha's hand was met with a cold stare.

# 4

'What would you like?' I asked Sujatha before placing my order at the counter.

We were at the café of the One⁰15 Marina club. I am a member of this prestigious club and often visit this place to have a few moments of relaxation.

It was around 5 p.m. on a Wednesday, and the place was sparsely populated. A few kids were cycling, and some others were in various stages of relaxation. We sat on one of the benches and gazed at the lovely blue waters of the ocean. The still-warm breeze messed up our hair, but it did not matter, to me at least.

I had called Sujatha the day after the tumultuous meeting in my clinic and asked her to join me here. A different setting which was more open would have probably put her at ease.

She seemed more relaxed than our previous meetings, although her awkwardness was still perceptible.

As the cold coffee soothed our parched throats, she said softly, 'I am sorry about last week.'

I reassured her, 'Don't worry about it, Sujatha. As a therapist, it is my job to meet people who may be going through difficult situations in their life. Please remove that thought from your mind.'

'Thank you, ma'am!' She seemed more relaxed now that the monkey was off her back.

'Would you want me to work with your daughter?' I asked her, wanting to be a little more assertive with my line of questioning.

'Most definitely,' she replied slowly but in an assured tone. 'I am surprised that I did not come to you earlier. I was telling my other daughter, Mala, who is in America, about you. She called me over the weekend and convinced me to take your services. Apparently, you have a lot of good references on the internet.'

'That's kind of her,' I said. A little appreciation makes everyone feel good.

I continued, 'Sujatha, if you want me to help Latha, this is what I want you to do. Please tell me everything about Latha which would help me understand her situation better. Can we do that today?'

She nodded her head, and I prepared myself to take some mental notes.

The family was originally from Cochin, a bustling city in the state of Kerala in India. After the initial years of marriage, they shifted to Chennai in early 2000, since her husband, Krishnan, an IT engineer, got a job there. Her daughters, Mala and Latha, started going to a premium school in Chennai. Her husband's role required him to travel a lot. The high stress associated with the job made him very irritable, and he took to drinking alcohol almost every night. In his inebriated state, he would take out his frustrations on Sujatha. They would end up having constant fights, and their relationships soured with each passing day. The situation worsened to such an extent that he would even abuse her physically. Unfortunately, her two daughters were witness to this family drama. Mala was old enough to comfort her mother, but Latha would get scared and run into her room every time there was a fracas. Ending the marriage legally would have been an easy option. However, Sujatha did not have the courage to take this decision, or more likely, she displayed a lot of courage by deciding to stay in the marriage and create a good life for her daughters.

She was from a conservative Brahmin family where traditions were revered, and she resorted to religion in these troubled times. She instilled a belief in her children that these rituals would lead to a better life. She would apply oil on their hair every night, insisting that they have a bath first thing in the morning and dress in traditional attire with their hair neatly braided and adorned with flowers. She would make them recite verses from the religious texts every evening. In fact, she even hired a tutor who would teach them the meaning of these texts. As was the practice in Chennai, where a typical Brahmin girl would be trained either in music or dance, she enrolled them in traditional Carnatic music class. While her own married life was going downhill with every passing day, she tried her best to shield her daughters from that trauma. Both the girls were good in academics and music. In 2013, Krishnan got a job at an MNC in Singapore, and the entire family shifted its base. Mala had just graduated, and she found a job in a local Singapore company. Latha was 16 and just out of school. She secured admission in one of the best international high schools in Singapore. Latha adjusted to the new surroundings quickly. Even in Singapore, Sujatha enrolled Latha in a music academy to ensure her connect with music. In 2015, Mala got married to Shyam, an IT professional who was her colleague at work and they migrated to America.

The sun had set, and the breeze was picking up. More people had filled the place, but I wanted to know more. Importantly, Sujatha was in a mood to talk.

'Please tell me more about Latha,' I said.

Sujatha seemed to be more comfortable with me now and showed an inclination to share more details. I listened intently for another hour.

It was way past 7 p.m. The ocean had gone dark, and the lights of the city were shining bright. I had just heard everything that Sujatha had to say, and my head was heavy. We sat in silence for a few minutes before I stood up and she followed suit. We continued to walk in silence away from the waters of the ocean.

# 5

'I will try' was Sujatha's response when I called her a couple of days ago and suggested that she get Latha to the clinic.

Sujatha seemed very sceptical by nature, and it would generally take a while to make her understand why I wanted certain things to be done. I have realised that it would be better to just tell her to do something rather than try and explain it.

'Come to my clinic with Latha at 11 a.m.' was my instruction to her. 'If she asks you why, tell her we will be meeting the lawyer.'

I was happy to see them in my clinic at fifteen minutes past 11 a.m.

The scene seemed to be a continuation of the other day, with Sujatha a bit wary and Latha a tad more aggressive.

After the initial pleasantries, I got down to business.

I looked at Latha and said, 'You mother has told me a lot about you. She has told me how much they love you. I am here to help you achieve your dreams. I am told that you are a very intelligent girl and that you will understand what I am saying.'

There was no response. The steely gaze continued to pierce me. Although unnerved, I did not shift my gaze from her eyes.

'What do you want to tell me?' I asked without referring to her by name.

She turned to Sujatha and growled, 'Why have you brought me here again?'

'I asked your mother to get you here,' I replied calmly.

'I don't want to talk to you, stupid lady,' she retorted.

Sujatha shuffled nervously in her chair and touched Latha's hand in an attempt to retrain her.

I ignored Sujatha's attempts and continued my conversation with Latha. 'I thought you are an intelligent girl and would realise that I am the only person who can help you. You have met so many therapists, but did they help? I am your last chance.'

Her gaze shifted down, which suggested that she was considering my point.

'I want to meet a lawyer,' she screamed.

'Yes, Latha, I will help you meet a lawyer.'

It was inadvertent. I had taken her name, and her response was immediate.

'*I am not Latha*,' she bawled. 'Can't you understand?'

'OK,' I said, maintaining my gentle tone. 'But I do know a lawyer who may be able to help you.'

She looked at me with her steely gaze, and I felt as if under scrutiny.

'Can you help me talk to a lawyer?' she said in a tone which seemed less like an enquiry and more like a command.

'I can do that but first let me know why,' I said.

And finally, she spoke something more, suggesting a change in her stance towards me.

'I want a passport for Jill,' she said brusquely.

'Jill?' I enquired 'Who is Jill?'

She did not respond and continued to stare at me. The curls on her forehead made her look more menacing. The silence was getting very discomforting, but I kept telling myself to remain calm.

'Latha, may I know who Jill is?' I asked, trying to be more forceful.

The anger in her seemed to now ooze out of every pore, and she gestured to make a move towards me. Sujatha held her hand tightly, which seemed to stop her advance.

'You don't understand, do you?' she howled again in between her heavy breathing.

'Latha, how can I help you if you don't tell me why you would like to meet a lawyer,' I tried to reason.

She screamed with her eyes closed and her feet again stomping the floor, '*I am not Latha.*'

She was shaking all over. Her breathing was now coming out as a groan. It was my turn to look at Sujatha.

Not getting any response from her, I asked, 'Oh sorry, who are you?'

'*I am Jane,* you stupid woman,' she yelled. 'Don't you understand?'

'OK, and who is Jill?' I prodded while still trying to maintain my composure.

'Can't you see, stupid woman?' she screamed. 'Jill is here.'

She was on boil. Her flaring eyes were piercing me, and I could see her trying to free her hand from her mother's grip. I was nervous, really nervous, both from her statement and from the perceived danger of physical harm. For a brief moment, I was lost for words.

I slowly gathered myself and took a few deep breaths 'Where is Jill?'

'I am Jill,' the soft voice answered.

A chill ran down my spine. It seemed like I was watching a horror movie and the spirit had just made an appearance.

Trying to find the right words, I stuttered, 'Yes ... I see that.'

'I want a lawyer to make a passport for me and Jill.' It was the coarse voice again.

I could feel my hands going numb as if hit by a bolt of lightning. I had experienced many difficult clients, but this was creepy. I needed some time to gather my nerves and really fathom what the girl was saying. I needed time to plan my next move.

'Fine,' I responded, trying to sound as calm as possible, 'I will speak to a lawyer and let you know. Would that be OK?'

There was no answer, but the piercing eyes did not leave me.

I turned to Sujatha. 'Sujatha, I will let you know when I have spoken to a lawyer. You can then inform Jane. Is that OK?'

'Sure, ma'am,' Sujatha responded with a nervous smile, and she stood up, sensing that I was keen to end the session.

After they left, I took a few deep breaths to calm myself. The coarse voice seemed to reverberate in the room, and I felt the need for some fresh air. I decided to walk back home.

We had taken some big steps today. Little did I realise that there was so much more to come.

I was in the café at the One⁰15 Marina club and gazed at the blue waters. Life can be so unpredictable. Here was a simple girl leading a normal life with plenty of dreams to achieve, and in the twinkle of an eye, everything seemed to be over.

My mind went back to the conversation with Sujatha at this very place. I wanted to play back her narration to pick up any strand which could help me get closer to understand this case. The thought of solving it was still some distance away.

Latha was a very obedient girl right from her childhood; very sincere in her studies and good at music, she was the typical South Indian Brahmin girl. She was generally very quiet and spent most of her time playing with her toys or reading books. Things started to change after they moved to Singapore. She was exposed to a more modern way of living. Her classmates were from different ethnic backgrounds and their association began to influence her. She became friendly with a boy from her class, Jaden. She was besotted by him. He was a much sought-after boy in high school. His handsome looks and his rockstar image meant that many girls would have a crush on him. Their world changed on Latha's 18ᵗʰ birthday. On the day which would normally be the most anticipated day in every girl's life, Latha's world came crashing down. She realised that Jaden was in a relationship with her best friend, Fiona. Latha was crushed. She locked herself in her room and refused to come out. Her mother's repeated attempts to make her understand from the other side of the door had no impact on her. Even Fiona's attempts to persuade her to come out and talk fell on deaf ears. It was Fiona who told Sujatha about Jaden and the events which had led to this situation. When the door finally opened a day later, Latha was a different girl. She stopped talking to anyone. She avoided school and her music class. She would hardly eat and generally confined herself to her room. Her mother's belief that this was a temporary issue proved otherwise when something bizarre came to light during her elder daughter's visit to Singapore.

I suddenly realised that it was getting dark. I checked my watch, which showed the time as 7 p.m. I headed back home. After dinner, I retired to my room and dimmed the lights. It was time to continue with the playback in my mind.

Mala and her husband Shyam had come on their annual visit. Unlike the past, when Latha would spend a lot of time with them, she refused to even meet them. She would be in her room, and even when she would come out a few times, she would ignore their presence. Sujatha was disturbed by this attitude and tried speaking with her gently at first and then even reprimanded her for this behaviour. It had no effect on Latha. In fact, during one of these conversations, Latha even warned Sujatha to stop speaking to them as well, or else she would have to face dire consequences. Sujatha was in a quandary. Her life was already in a mess with her failed marriage and this latest turn of events was becoming too much for her. She would cry in her room and pray to her God, seeking His divine help. The change in environment was not lost on Mala. After spending a few days at Shyam's parents' home in India, she travelled back to Singapore to be with her mother.

It was Mala who noticed it first.

Mala was not able to sleep one night. As she was passing by Latha's room, she heard some voices from inside. She first thought it must be coming from Latha's mobile phone, but when she strained her ears to the door, she realised they were human voices. She tried to decipher what was being spoken but could not. It was more of a mumble, but she could definitely identify two voices. The next morning, she knocked on Latha's door, but there was no response. She asked her mother whether Latha had a friend over the previous night, but it had been weeks since Latha had even spoken to any of her friends. Mala sensed something was wrong. She stayed awake the following night, and soon enough, she heard the voices from within Latha's room. There were two distinct voices; one was very coarse, and the other was feeble, but she could not make out what was being said. This happened intermittently every night and made Mala realise that something was seriously wrong with Latha. Her attempts to know more from Latha fell on deaf ears. Latha refused to even look at Mala, let alone speak to her. It was then that Mala suggested Sujatha seek professional help. With Mala back in the US, Sujatha took Latha to many therapists but to no avail. They even visited a psychiatrist, but apart from putting her under severe medication, nothing changed.

With Mala back in the US, an indifferent husband, a failed marriage, and a daughter who was probably going crazy, life couldn't be any worse for Sujatha. It was in this condition that we had met at the coffee house.

Our bitter experiences are stored as memories in some corner of our mind. We would rather not visit these dark places in fear of spoiling our present. However, it is proven that the better way to get rid of these bitter memories is to face them without any fear and consciously get rid of them in such a way that they are no longer significant. Of course, this is easier said than done.

## 6

That meeting occupied my mind space for most of the next few days. As was my practice, after a few intense therapy sessions, I would always engage in some activity where I could be totally absorbed. These activities are not only therapeutic for my clients but were a wonderful stressbuster for me. In fact, I have never recommended therapy to a client without first experiencing it myself.

Yoga therapy involves self-expression based on Indian mythology. The best projections are of Lord Shiva in various forms of yoga and dances depicting his moods. Ancient Vedic scriptures have given vigorous combination of yoga and dance to achieve positive mental health, which is the joyful union of mind and body. Dance and yoga have long been described as two rivers stemming from the same source. In their simplest definitions, yoga and dance can be reduced to breathing with movement or breath-guided movement. One major identity that links dance and yoga is the concept of *prana*, or life force, that stems from breath. The yogi and the dancer, however, have a closer relationship with prana and their own breathing habits. The major difference between yoga and dance is the focus. While we do yoga from a place inside the body and mind—and that's where the focus should stay throughout practice—it's never about achieving the 'perfect pose' or wanting to force the body into an asana or a particular posture. Dance, on the other hand, has its focus on the outward performance and aesthetics.

Yoga transported me to a different world, where I was free from pressures and expectations of people around me. It created an invisible shield which protected me from all the negative energies.

Back in my clinic, a more rejuvenated me made a call to Sujatha and fixed an appointment for Tuesday of the following week.

# 7

When she walked into my clinic, she seemed a different person from whom I had met earlier. She looked ragged. Her clothes and hair were all over the place, her face seemed weary, and there was a huge cut next to her left eye.

'What happened?' was my first question upon seeing her in this state as I got up from my chair and stepped forward.

'I … I fell down in the washroom,' she replied with a sheepish look.

'Are you sure you are fine?' I enquired, worried about her condition.

'I am fine. Thanks!' was her response. Something was not right, but I decided not to probe further for now.

'Sujatha, be comfortable and let me know when we can start talking.'

She broke down and between her sobs murmured, 'Life is tough, ma'am. I need your help.'

I waited for a few seconds and then held a glass of water and a box of tissues for her.

'Here take this and let's find a solution to your present situation,' I assured her.

She took a few tissues to wipe her tears, drank the water, and slowly reached some semblance of control. She started twiddling her fingers again.

'Latha's condition is getting worse. She has hardly spoken a word in the past few days. She does not come out of the room. She keeps talking to herself. She gets violent when I try to talk to her,' Sujatha confided nervously.

I decided that it was time to probe further on a few leads. I would normally want to know about my client's past from the client himself or herself, but this case was different. I had to understand more details about Latha from Sujatha, and there was a possibility that her version may not include specifics which may only be known to Latha. I had to be very precise with my line of questioning.

'Sujatha, did you notice anything different about Latha before the incident with her boyfriend?'

She took a moment.

'Latha was always studious and a very obedient girl. I don't remember too many instances when I had to scold her,' she recollected.

'Can you narrate any incident when you had to scold her?' I asked.

'It was silly,' she said as a smile escaped her lips 'She must have been about 10 years old. Mala won the singing competition in their school and got a trophy. Latha had also taken part in that competition in her age category but did not win. When we came home, she held on to the trophy and would not let anyone touch it. She would scream, "This is my trophy" when anyone even spoke about it. Mala was also young, and she wanted the trophy on her study table. They had a huge fight, and Mala had to grab the trophy from her. Latha was crying the whole day and refused to eat. Both Krishnan and I scolded her. I remember Krishnan even slapped her a few times to bring her under control.'

'What was she angry about?' I prodded.

'About not winning the trophy, I guess,' she replied after some thought.

'Sujatha, I want you to think.' I leaned towards her. 'Was she angry about not winning the trophy or that everyone was appreciating her sister?'

The shifting of her gaze suggested that she was searching for that incident in her memory bank.

'Can you go back to that incident and recollect your reactions and those of people around you,' I suggested.

She thought aloud. 'I remember many teachers came and appreciated Mala and spoke highly of her. In fact, the principal came and personally congratulated her and called her an asset to the school. Krishnan and I were also happy and showered praises on her.'

'And what about Latha?' I asked. 'Did she congratulate her sister?'

'I can't remember … but I don't think she did,' Sujatha said as she strained her memory. 'You are right. Probably, she was upset because she did not get the appreciation.'

'And what made you say that?' I probed further.

That question probably opened a line of thought as her eyes widened.

'Now that you have mentioned it, I think you are right. I have seen her sulk every time we would appreciate Mala for something. At that time, I thought it was because she was a kid. But now, it seems different …'

Her words trailed away

'Was Mala good in her studies?'

'Yes, she was. She would always be the top ranker in her class,' Sujatha replied.

'And what about her singing?' I asked.

'Well, Mala was good at everything she did. She was gifted,' she said.

'So, she would also receive a lot of appreciation from people, including you?'

'Hmmm,' she replied.

'Sujatha, some people are very sensitive about their ego and self-esteem. They need constant reassurances from people around them. Things can get bad when they see others getting the appreciation and none coming their way. They feel ignored. They feel let down. In this moment of weakness, they don't look at the practical side. They don't try and understand that the appreciation may be justified. When this happens over a period of time, they start questioning their own abilities. They start feeling worthless.'

Sujatha was listening intently.

'These are assumptions at the moment, but I need your help to understand more such possibilities,' I explained.

'Did Latha have a lot of friends?' I asked.

'Not many. She was not very social. Her world was confined to her books and her free time was also spent at home.'

'Can you remember some of her friends?'

She thought for a moment and said, 'She had a good friend Raji in her school days. They would spend a lot of time together. They were very close. After her tenth grade, Raji moved to a different part of the city for her high school, and I have not seen them together after that.'

'Can you describe Raji?' I enquired.

Seeing her blank expression, I rephrased my question.

'Was Raji also studious? Was she good in other activities? What was her family background? These are the things that I want to know,' I clarified.

'Raji was an all-rounder. Not exceptional in studies, but she would be involved in many activities. I think she was also the school head girl in their ninth grade. She was beautiful and carried herself well. She was always well dressed,' Sujatha said, sharing her thoughts. 'And one more thing: she was already riding a scooter when she was in tenth grade. Latha used to keep telling me about it.'

'OK. What about your time in Singapore?' I asked.

'She did make some friends in her high school. She was excited about seeing the boys and girls from different cultures. She would tell me how their habits are so different from ours.'

'What about Jaden?' I enquired.

'Jaden was her classmate in school. She would talk about him. He has also come home a few times. They had a common friend, Fiona. Fiona would also come home regularly, and they have had a few sleepovers.'

'Can you describe Jaden?' I asked, ticking off my questions one by one.

'Well, I don't know much about him. I have seen him a few times. Long blond hair, and he would wear very weird clothes, like those pop stars you see on TV. I remember, I was shocked when I saw him once with his ears pierced and decorated with gold studs,' she recalled.

'Did Latha share anything about her fondness for Jaden?' I asked.

'No, she never shared very private details about anyone. Even in the case of Raji, I only knew some details from Raji herself.'

'How did you know about their relationship?' I asked.

'From her second year of high school, she changed a lot. She would stand in front of the mirror a lot. She would want to shop for clothes. She was more particular about what she wore. I had seen a similar change in Mala, so I related it to teenage fantasies. Also, we were in a different country which was so much more modern as compared to Chennai. But I never suspected anything going on between her and Jaden,' she confessed.

'Can you share more details about her 18th birthday?' I enquired since that seemed to be a defining day.

'She had planned a dinner with her friends. I did not know who would be there, but she had asked for S$100 from me. In fact, her father had a showdown with her about the time she was spending with her friends and for neglecting her studies. I wanted her to enjoy her big day and gave her the money without the knowledge of her father. She left for her school in the morning, and I did not hear from her during the entire day. I tried calling her in the afternoon, but she did not answer. I tried informing Krishnan, but he was busy with some clients. I called her school in the evening, but the office did not know about her whereabouts. I remember, she came home around 10 p.m. She looked really angry. She did not speak to anyone and went straight to her room, banging the door shut behind her. Krishnan was livid and shouted at her to come out. He started banging her door from outside. She did not open the door at all. In his anger, Krishnan hurt his hand while banging the door, and he needed medical attention. As usual, he removed his frustrations on me that night.'

She fell silent as her train of thoughts had led her in a different direction.

'And that's what he did to you last evening as well?' I asked, seizing the opportunity to probe further on her facial injury.

The statement seemed to touch a raw nerve. She broke down uncontrollably. I had to get up and comfort her. She stood up and embraced me tightly while the tears flowed incessantly.

I just held her without saying a word. The lady had gone through hell and had probably relived that hell again as she would have done with the other therapists she may have consulted.

That outburst also gave a clue to her facial injury. I made a mental note to deal with it once I make some headway in this case.

I let her calm down, gave her a cup of tea, and when she felt better, bid her goodbye, promising to call her in a couple of days.

I had drawn many inferences based on what I had heard from Sujatha. I now had to deal with Latha.

I came up with a plan.

# 8

It was a very wet day. I would have preferred to remain at home, but I had my session with Sujatha. While I do know that we should not let the weather decide our mood, the gloomy, grey sky sometimes betrays these thoughts.

I reached my clinic early and had a hot cup of green tea. I selected the book *Discover Your Destiny,* by Robin Williams, from my bookshelf and engrossed myself in the inspirational pages. I had just reached the page where the great coach had spent a day with his client when there was a knock on my door.

Sujatha peeped in with a polite request. 'May I come in?'

'Of course, Sujatha.' I stood up to receive her.

She was more organised today. She was wearing an off-white saree, which, with the pleated hair and bindi, completed her traditional look.

As she made herself comfortable, I asked, 'How are you today?'

'I am OK,' she replied in the soft, husky voice that I was so used to now.

'Do you want to share anything with me,' I asked.

'Things are the same,' she said in a voice which conveyed a sense of resignation.

'I have a plan,' I jumped onto the subject.

She was an eager listener, as I explained to her what I had in mind. I reiterated every point to ensure her understanding and concurrence. She had a couple of questions which confirmed her attention. Once I was done, I looked at her for a response.

She sat in silence, gazing at the floor as she ran the idea in her head. Once she was done, she looked up and gave me a gentle nod which conveyed acceptance but did not indicate confidence.

'What do you have to say?' I asked her, wanting to get her doubts clarified.

She responded, 'It will be difficult, but I will try. Since the last few months, I have not had a conversation with her. She generally dismisses me or refuses to talk.'

'Sujatha, in life, we encounter many situations when we fear treading a path and accept other choices as the only ones we have. However, we have to realise that the other choices are nothing but a mere ignorance of the situation. It does not take you forward. This is one such moment. What we discussed may be difficult but may be the only way to move from where we are. In what direction, I am not sure, but move we will. Not doing it may seem an easy option, but then, we are likely to remain where we are, and that I am sure of. That is not solving the problem, is it?' I asked the rhetorical question and allowed her time to reflect.

'You are right,' she said after a few minutes of silence.

'If you are fine with it, I would like to do a therapy for you to help you feel calm and more self-confident. May I?' I asked.

'Sure,' she replied, eager to get whatever help she could find.

Sujatha was on the therapy chair for the rest of the session, and it was a more assured person who left the clinic that day. She had to don a very different avatar than what she was, and it would require more than just willpower to see this through. A better life at the end of this ordeal was the hope she carried.

I was nervous since it was the first time I was getting therapy done through someone else. That was the only way I could reach the real Latha. I was hoping that Sujatha would be able to bring her to a state from where I could take over.

The mission had begun.

## 9

For Sujatha, it was a new day. She could see the silver lining among the grey clouds in her head. She was happy that Krishnan was travelling and would not be back for another week. Once she reached home, she settled herself and knocked on the door of Latha's room.

'Can I come in?' she asked loudly.

There was no answer.

Sujatha entered anyway. The room was dark as the shades were drawn and the lights were not switched on. Sujatha switched the lamp on her study table to get some light. She was lying on the bed. Her face was not visible behind the long tresses which were spread over the front of her face, giving her an eerie look in the dim light.

Sujatha sat near her and gently held her hand. It was rather cold.

'How are you doing?' Sujatha asked as she slowly moved the hair to one side revealing her face.

Her eyes were wide open—in fact, wider than normal—and they were staring at her.

Sujatha recited her prayers in her head to calm herself.

'I was preparing for dinner. What would you like to have?' Sujatha asked with a nervous smile.

'You know what I like?' she replied in a coarse voice.

Sujatha knew what to do.

'Pasta?' Sujatha asked. 'I know you like pasta … Jane,' Sujatha said, firing her first salvo.

There was no response. Sujatha tried other ways of starting a conversation, but the teenager was in no mood.

Sujatha recollected Preeti's advice: 'Be patient. And be persistent.' She decided to try again that evening.

It started raining very heavily that evening. Bursts of thunder broke the eerie silence in the Nair house. Sujatha had initially felt relieved at Krishnan's absence, but in the situation she was in, she probably would have felt more assured in the presence of another person, however indifferent that person's sensitivities.

Sujatha was scared. She made the pasta she had promised and took it to her daughter's room. The room was even darker now, and the light from the window cast shadows on the wall behind the bed that she was sitting on. Sujatha quickly put on the lights and reminded herself that it was her daughter on the bed.

'Look what I have made for you Jane,' she said slowly.

She was sitting in a crouched position with her head between her knees. Hearing Sujatha, she looked up.

Sujatha set two bowls on the study table and said softly, 'Come, let's have some lovely pasta' and took a bite from her own bowl. 'Yummy, this is so tasty.'

She got up from the bed and took the few steps to the table. The smell of the pasta drew her to the food, and the taste made her devour the contents. It had been many months since Sujatha had seen her eat so well. After the dinner, Sujatha closed the kitchen for the night, then came back to her daughter's room and sat near her.

'Did you enjoy the food?' Sujatha said as she held her hand. She smiled.

Sensing the opportunity, Sujatha moved to a position next to her and laid a pillow behind her own back and rested on it. This could take a long time.

Sujatha gently took her daughter's head and laid it on her lap. She did not resist.

'I realised that we have not had a conversation for a long time Jane,' Sujatha said lovingly, 'and I am responsible for that. I have been busy with the house—with Mala, with your father—and have not spent sufficient time with you. I am going to change all that now. I know my baby needs me.'

Sujatha felt a lump in her throat as the realisation dawned on her about the truth in what she had just said. Her daughter's face was turned down, but her hands tightened their grip on Sujatha's lap. After a few minutes of silence, during which Sujatha was running her fingers through her hair, she finally spoke.

'Jill, I'm going to talk to you loudly so that Amma can hear.' The coarse voice was speaking. 'I want to ask Amma if she wants to tell us what she has already spoken to the lady we met the other day.'

That was sudden but was definitely what Sujatha wanted.

'Amma will tell you,' Sujatha said and slowly narrated her conversations with Preeti.

When she finished, the coarse voice spoke. 'Let me tell you the truth, Jill. Why I want to go to that lady is because I want to find out what to do, since there seem to be two people in this body—I want to get proof of this so that I can prove it to other people as well. Maybe the two people seem to be twins. Maybe something has happened to us.'

Sujatha listened nervously.

The coarse voice continued, 'I want to talk about something interesting so Amma does not get bored. Did you love anyone?'

Finally, the softer voice spoke. 'Yes, only one person—Jaden in upper school.'

Sujatha was petrified now. This was the first time she had heard her daughter speak in this other voice, which was so different. This was also the first time that she was probably so close to a conversation happening between two people who had been living in her house but who were not known to her.

She remembered Dr Preeti telling her to remain calm at all times. She started reciting her prayers again.

'Are you sure you loved him?' It was the coarse voice.

'Yes.'

'Do you love him now?'

'No' was the answer from the soft voice.

The coarse voice continued, 'Jill, you and me don't want to get into trouble with Amma, Appa, or with Dr Preeti for being what we are—two people in the same body. I am going to tell Amma the secrets. We should find out if we are something rare in this world. It's extremely difficult for you that I am sharing the secrets with Amma. I don't know whom to go to.'

'Jaden seems to be kind of stupid—he does not seem to understand that you are beautiful … He goes to Fiona. I hate Fiona Fussy. Jill, right now, you are very nervous that I am telling your secrets to Amma. Jill, I should comfort you. Jill, it's OK. I am comforting you. Why don't you talk?'

The soft voice spoke again. 'My name is Jill. I am two … two … 21 years old. I don't know about my sexuality. I need help. My m-m … mind seems to carry on without me. I liked the boy called A … A … Arnab in grade 2. In grade 3, I liked Ravi and M-M … Malik. In grade 5, I liked Sam and also Kapil. In grade 8, I liked M-M … Muthu but not much. In grade 10, the same two people. Oh yes, in grade 10, there was another guy called P-P-Patrick. In grade 11, I liked Jaden, and he was the best …'

Sujatha noticed the distinct stammer in her voice.

This was the first of many strange conversations that Sujatha was part of over the next few days. After every conversation, she would call me, and I would suggest next steps. I kept reassuring Sujatha that she had to tread very carefully to maintain this communication, although nothing being said was making any sense to her.

The coarse voice would always start talking on some random subject.

'The real reason why I wanted to go out of the school is that I wanted to go harder on you, Jill. I wanted to keep you safe by doing all kinds of things. The worst thing that happened was him.'

The coarse voice would then urge the softer voice to speak.

The soft voice would provide an equally random response. 'Amma, Jane told me some th-th-things. She seems to think that there are t-t-two people in this body. But what is the truth? Maybe someone should tell us. Someone should t-t-tell us what is really happening. I feel that I am always losing. It h-h-hurts. I am in physical pain. I don't know what to do.'

Invariably, she would be in tears during her narration.

'Maybe, I need to start from sc-sc-scratch to learn about how to live. Maybe I don't want to have another p-p-person in the body. Maybe I do. I seem to hide from the sa-sa-sadist psycho rascal called God who wants to put me in h-h-hell. He wants to hurt me—this God guy. He is like a mo-mo-monster on my back. He is spying on me. He is watching me and ju-ju-judging me and forcing me to go to hell. Maybe I don't know the difference between right and wrong. Why is God following me around? Maybe God is following me. I feel like I am getting b-b-blackmailed by God. He is not allowing me to be m-m-myself. Jane taught me all kinds of things. Now I don't know what's going to happen to me. Maybe I don't know. Maybe I feel like cr-cr-crying, even though I can't cry. Maybe I relate to the song called 'What Now?' by Ri-Ri-Rihanna.'

'I am hurting badly—emotionally m-m-mentally, spiritually, and physically. Why would they give me a b-b-blood test? What if Jane and you all decide to to-to-torture me? Why didn't the social worker, m-m-my family, friends, and relatives help me? What am I really like? I don't know. I don't know what I want and what I don't want? Earlier, I felt I could not m-m-move ... How I would be? I would be just making no-no-noises—just wanting to scream. Everything seems weird. Amma, you seem to think I got bullied that's why I am having problems. I feel that people don't know how to talk to me. I want to have a bo-bo-boyfriend.'

Sujatha couldn't wait to share these details with me. Importantly, she had also done something that I had suggested. She had recorded the conversations on her mobile phone.

Sujatha shared the audio files with me over the internet. Once I was in the clinic, I told my assistant that I did not wish to be disturbed, and in the total silence of the therapy room, I played the audio recordings. As the conversation played out, it could be easily mistaken for two girls having an innocent chat. However, when I could put it in context and visualise the scene in the Nair house, where this scene was playing out, I could feel a chill down my spine. I actually turned up the temperature of the air conditioner. I even had to rewind some parts and hear them again to decipher what was being said and to draw some inference from them.

The few days that I followed this routine are etched in my memory due to the deep impact it caused.

## 10

Sujatha came to the clinic, accompanied by Latha. They looked like any other normal mother and daughter. It was a pity that circumstances had led to the current situation that they found themselves in. However, in the dark clouds that they seem to be surrounded by, I could see the flicker of light.

Once they had taken their seats, I addressed Latha.

'Hello, Latha. How are you?' I asked, wanting to see the response.

She kept staring at me.

'Are you Latha?' I probed, trying to elicit a response.

There was none.

I turned to Sujatha and said, 'Sujatha, you were telling me how much you love Jane and Jill. I am here to help. Please tell them.'

'Don't you understand?' the coarse voice shouted.

I was startled with the sudden interjection but happy that I got a response.

'Hello, Jane. I was waiting for you,' I said.

'Where is the lawyer?' she questioned.

'I need to tell the lawyer about you and Jill. Your mother has told me everything that you have asked her to share. What do you want to tell me?'

'I don't want to tell you anything,' she shouted menacingly.

'Your Amma tells me that you like singing,' I persisted.

'Don't you understand? I don't like singing. Jill likes to sing.' She sounded even angrier.

'That's wonderful. Jill, can you sing?' I asked.

'Are you crazy? I am Jane, and I don't like singing,' she said.

'Can you ask Jill to sing?' I asked.

There was a pause, and then the coarse voice said, 'Jill doesn't want to sing.'

I said, 'I have been speaking to a lawyer, and he has asked me to get all the details of Jane and Jill. If Jill doesn't speak, I will not be able to help.'

'I want to sing,' the soft voice spoke for the first time, 'but I need permission from Jane.'

'Please go ahead and get the permission,' I said now that I had managed to get both of them speaking to me.

'Jane has given me permission,' the soft voice said and started singing.

She had a melodious voice, but there was no rhythm.

'That was wonderful, Jill,' I said after she had sung a few lines of a classical song.

Sujatha had a smile on her face. She had possibly heard her daughter sing for the first time in many months, albeit in a very different voice.

'Jill, you have a sweet voice,' I said. 'Unless you sing more often, how will others know about it? How will they appreciate you?' I thought of an idea which would help her come closer to the mainstream. 'Why don't you recite the prayers every evening at your home? Will you do that?'

She replied softly, 'I will do that, but I need permission from Jane.'

We waited.

After a few seconds, she spoke again 'Jane has given me permission.'

'That's wonderful, Jill. I am so happy for you,' I assured her with all the excitement I could muster.

'What do you like to do, Jane?' I asked, eager to engage with the other personality.

There was silence. Although her anger had subsided, her fists were still clenched tightly, and her upright sitting position suggested that she was still not comfortable.

I tried different ways to make her talk, but nothing worked. I let them leave after some time. Before leaving, I told Sujatha to encourage Latha to recite the prayers every evening. I also asked her to try and have their conversations outside her bedroom. I needed to get her out of that room more often.

## 11

The sound of the alarm woke me. It took a minute for me to orient myself, probably the result of a dream that I may have been in the middle of. As I stretched myself, my eyes fell on the painting which adorned my bedroom wall, where the lovely landscape of a flower valley was getting its first light from the rising sun. At that moment, I got my answer to the question which was vexing me since last night. I jumped out of my bed and made some quick notes. I was ready for the next session.

Unlike my usual practice of having my sessions at my clinic or a location which was ideal for the situation in hand, I decided to visit the Nair home.

The Nairs lived in one of the modern apartment complexes, which are now a common feature of modern Singapore. The complex had a swimming pool and a play area for children, surrounded by tall buildings on either side. The flat itself was typically South Indian, with a four-foot Natraj statue welcoming visitors as soon as they entered. The smell of incense filled the house. Sujatha greeted me and led me to their living room, which was moderately furnished. I made myself comfortable on the sofa while Sujatha went into the kitchen and came back with a glass of water.

The initial formalities done, I moved on to business.

Sujatha apprised me of the developments of the previous two days. Latha was very social on the first day, and she even chanted the prayers that evening. However, she was back into her shell the next day. Sujatha was disappointed with this, but to me, it seemed normal.

I asked her, 'Sujatha, you had mentioned in one of our earlier conversations that Latha was going to an art class before her illness.'

Sujatha responded, 'Yes, I had enrolled her in the Pearl Academy of Fine Arts, where she was learning to paint.'

'Was she enjoying it?' I asked.

She replied, 'Well … not really.'

'You had also mentioned that Mala was good at painting. Am I right?' I enquired.

'Yes, she was very good.' She pointed to a painting on the wall in the dining area. 'That's her painting.'

'That's perfect,' I said, feeling a sense of elation.

Sujatha did not understand, but I had my plan ready.

'Can we speak to Latha?' I asked.

Sujatha went inside the house and after a few minutes came back with Latha. She seemed like any other normal girl today. Her hair was well oiled and neatly combed with a pleat.

'Hello, Jane,' I asked, guessing the personality that might want to communicate with me.

'Why have you come here?' was the coarse response.

'I was passing by and came to visit you,' I said and added. 'You look very nice today.'

Pulling her hair, she grumbled, 'I hate this oily hair. I don't know how Jill can like it.'

'It makes you look nice, and …'

I was about to complete when I realised I could use this situation in a better way.

'Jane, it looks like Jill is doing a lot of things that she likes doing. Why don't you do something that only you like?'

'What is that?' the coarse voice asked.

'Painting,' I exclaimed, waiting for a positive response—and I got it.

'I like painting,' she said, sounding excited. 'I want to do it.'

'That's fantastic,' I said. 'Your mother told me you were good. I will ask your mother to enrol you to an arts academy.'

The suggestion spurred her into a good mood, and Jane shared some more details of her life with Jill.

In every case, there is always a moment when something clicks. From that moment onwards, the client therapy took a turn for the better.

This was probably the defining moment in Latha's case.

## 12

There was a big change in Latha over the next three months. She started going to the arts academy more regularly. She also rejoined her music classes. Although she still had terrible mood swings and frequent bouts of bad temper, it was the periods in between which indicated a change for the better. Sujatha was playing her part very well. She would pamper Latha with food and some motherly love. I would also appreciate her for the smallest of things and play along with her.

Now that I had managed to clearly identify the two personalities, it was time for the next step. For that, I needed to be more assertive with her.

That day when Latha came to the clinic with Sujatha, she started singing.

I asked, 'That's a nice song. Who is singing?'

Her expressions changed, and anger enveloped her face.

'Can't you see it's me singing?' she retorted.

I asked in an equally loud voice, 'Who are you?'

She did not hold back and continued, 'You don't understand. I am Latha.'

That was an unexpected response, which took me by surprise and also made Sujatha sit up. It had been a while since she had heard her daughter's name.

I gathered my thoughts. 'Oh, yes. That's right. Then where are Jane and Jill?'

She looked at me in anger. 'You don't understand. There are two people living inside me.'

That was a huge acknowledgement

I asked, 'Are they living with you?'

'Did I say "living with me"?' she retorted 'What kind of a psychotherapist are you? You are not qualified. You can't even remember this.'

'Very sorry, Latha. I was—' I tried to make amends but was cut short.

'You don't even know English,' and she turned to her mother. 'She does not understand what I am saying. Why have you brought me here?'

'I am sorry. I did not understand correctly. Please, tell me again.'

She was in no mood to accept my apology. 'You are wasting my time,' she said and stood up in readiness to leave.

Sujatha held her close and cajoled her to calm down and listen to me.

When I sensed she had calmed down, I made another attempt. 'What were you saying, Latha?'

She looked at me in anger. 'There are two people living inside me.'

'OK,' I said without any reaction.

'Does it not mean anything to you? Are you OK with it?' she retorted.

This was going nowhere. I had to change the subject.

'I heard that Jane is doing very well in her arts course. Have you brought her painting?' I asked.

Sujatha removed her paintings from the folder she was carrying.

'These are so nice,' I said. 'You are so talented, Jane.'

I could see her expressions changing. She was listening intently.

'And what about Jill's singing? I am eager to listen to her songs,' I said, shifting my attention on the other personality.

The next thirty minutes were spent going through each painting and listening to songs. Sujatha and I ensured that we applauded every action.

I was happy that we had reached a stage where Latha was emerging from the shadows of the two personalities which had otherwise engulfed her.

## 13

Sujatha seems so much happier these days. Her troubles with her husband continue, but the improvement in Latha has lifted a huge burden off her shoulders. She has been putting a lot of effort into maintaining communication with Latha, keeping her patience through Latha's tantrums, and taking her to classes while also taking care of the house. To add to her already busy schedule, I suggested that she enrol Latha in a pottery class. Pottery is a wonderful activity for improving motor control, and I felt Latha needed it to improve her concentration as well. Convinced with my methods, she has now hired a maid who accompanies Latha to all her classes.

Jane would say, 'I don't like pottery,' and I would ask Jill to seek Jane's permission every time she had to go to the pottery class.

During these past months, I had been trying to narrow down the personalities to one personality, so I was making her do things that Latha would like but through two different people. I was making her feel appreciated. I was making her recognise her own talents. I was trying to make her believe in herself. I was trying to make her feel loved.

Since she had been on medication for more than a year, I asked Sujatha to visit the psychiatrist again and change her medicines. She did that, and the reduced dosage helped reduce Latha's mood swings. She was more alert now and could be seen outside her room more often.

It's been six months now since I met Sujatha at the cafe, and Latha has reached a more balanced state of mind in her road to recovery. She mingles with people. She goes for her classes. She does not talk to herself anymore. Jane and Jill are still there, but they are not aggressive. They seem to coexist.

I am happy that she has started becoming part of the crowd. She is going to places on her own. She would come to my clinic on her own, normally on her way home from her art class. She would come and show me her paintings. She would show me the painting that she was working on that day.

I would ask, 'Who has done this?'

She would show one part of the picture and say Jill had done this and another part that Jane had done. I am now working to reach a stage where the whole painting is either done by Jane or Jill.

I know this will take time, but I am confident of the direction I need to take.

Well, it's been one of my most intriguing cases.

Scary ... well, not anymore.

# CHAPTER 3

# PSYCHOTIC MEDITATION

## 1

I was in the lounge of Changi International Airport waiting for my flight to Mumbai. I was really looking forward to this journey, as it would be my first chance to visit the Global Vipassana Pagoda in India. As a Vipassana practitioner, I would have the privilege to spend a day in meditation at this renowned centre. I was bubbling with enthusiasm just like a child who is looking forward to her visit to a toy store.

As I settled down in the Singapore Airlines flight, a charming old lady came towards me with a big smile and greeted, 'Good evening' as she occupied the seat next to me.

I smiled and reciprocated.

She was fair-complexioned and plump, with a twinkle in her eye. She was wearing a very traditional dress, which I knew was the traditional Burmese dress, the *longyi*. The travels with my husband had taken me to many countries and one of them was Myanmar. Longyi is a wraparound skirt worn by men and women in that country.

Presuming she was from that country, I said, *'Nei kaurn thala,'* which was a common greeting in Myanmar.

Her face lit up even more, and she turned towards me. *'s ngya s nyya myanmar k nay parsalarr?'*

That was beyond my limited comprehension of the Burmese language, so I quickly reverted to known territory.

'I have lived in Myanmar for some time and hence know only a few words,' I admitted sheepishly in English.

'Oh, that's lovely. I am from Myanmar,' she responded. 'My name is Hla. What's yours?'

I introduced myself, and we began conversing.

My husband's company in Singapore posted him in Myanmar for seven years, from 1997 to 2004. The family shifted base to the country with a rich heritage. The people still followed most of the traditions passed on through centuries. However, many years of misrule had impoverished the country, and there was a big divide between the very rich and the poor. Away from the busy schedules of Singapore, Myanmar gave me the opportunity to do things that I had always wanted to do. I would play tennis in the morning and even got an opportunity to deliver psychology lectures at Dagon University. In a short time, I could build a good reputation, and I was given the responsibility of setting up the Psychology Equipment Lab at the university.

Thanks to my husband's work, I got an opportunity to meet a number of government officials and ambassadors. These interactions gave me a wider perspective about Myanmar and the world. My work at the university was getting recognised, and it resulted in an invitation from an elderly lady, whom I had never met before. Little did I know that this invitation would influence my life to the extent that it did.

The lady was the aunt of Mrs Usha Narayanan, the wife of the then president of India, Mr K. R. Narayanan. She was very happy with my work even more so because no foreign national had created such an impact in the university before. To my surprise, she called her famous niece in India right in the middle of our conversation and spoke highly about me.

The cordial meeting with the elderly lady resulted in an invitation from the wife of the president of India, to visit her in New Delhi.

When I did visit the Rashtrapati Bhavan, I was humbled by the graciousness of the president and his wife. The two-hour meeting extended to four hours of discussion on a wide variety of topics. The first lady gifted me with books from her collection, including her own *Sweet Memories*.

That meeting would remain etched in my memory forever.

The meeting opened many doors for me, and back in Myanmar, I was appointed the president of the UN newsletter. I took the initiative to publish a travel book, highlighting the glorious history of the country and how it can be a wonderful tourist destination.

My days became busier as meetings with government officials and ambassadors dotted my calendar. There were more invitations for lunches and dinners. In fact, I remember that I had put on 10 kg during that period. My husband took a liking to Mohinga, a traditional Burmese dish, and every day, someone would deliver this lovely dish to our house.

I even got an opportunity to meet the Burmese leader Miss Aung San Suu Kyi at one of the state dinners.

On the request of a government minister, I even took over the reins of a local orphanage. Spending time with the twelve kids in the orphanage, caring for them, teaching them, and sharing stories with them was therapeutic, and those were some of the best days of my life. I even bought a house and donated it to the orphanage so the children could have a decent place of shelter. I recollect that I had convinced my husband's company to hire two of the older boys from the orphanage.

It felt good to share these lovely memories with my co-passenger.

'You are Indian?' she asked after listening to my story.

I replied, 'I was born there but now live in Singapore.'

'When you lived in Myanmar, did you visit the Shiva temple in Sagiang?' she asked.

'Oh, yes,' I replied. 'I had the opportunity to go there a few times.'

'I like it,' she said. 'Very nice. Very spiritual. I go there often.'

The Shiva temple was a very old structure and frequented not only by the Indians who lived in Myanmar but also by the locals. It was more a spiritual retreat than a religious one and hence attracted people from different faiths. I had the good fortune to visit the temple on Maha Shivaratri, a festival of Lord Shiva. The large crowd of devotees were chanting 'Om Namah Shivay' in unison. As I sat at a distance and absorbed the divine sounds, I was transported to a different plane.

As my flight began its journey to the land of my birth, the chants of 'Om Namah Shivay' reverberated in my head, and that moment brought back memories of someone who had been a part of my life. My mind turned its attention to Kevin.

## 2

'I thought this cafe was renowned for its service.'

The loud voice distracted me, and I turned my head in the direction from where it originated. The year was 2011, and I was at Freshly Brewed, a café in Tanglin centre, back home in Singapore. I would normally spend some time here to read my notes and prepare for my sessions. This was one of those days.

The owner of the rather loud voice was a gentleman, very thin, tall, fair, Oriental in his features. If not for the scowl on his face at this moment, he might have been labelled handsome.

'Sir, we cannot move the furniture,' the young attendant was trying to explain.

'What's the point of having these plug points if there is no light here?' the gentleman continued his loud tirade. 'How can I work in this light?'

The young attendant seemed flustered and was at a loss for words. 'Sir, please try to understand' was all he could muster.

'If you cannot arrange for some lights here, I would like to sit on one of the sofas over there,' he shouted, pointing in the direction of the seating area where I was.

The entire café was now disturbed, and I could see some people even walking out. The outburst was completely out of place and showed the person in very poor light. Partly because I had almost finished my coffee and more so out of pity for the attendant, I got up from the sofa I was sitting on.

I raised my hand to let the agitated individual know that I was addressing him. 'Sir, hello,' I said, trying to get his attention.

When he finally looked in my direction, I said, 'You can take my seat here.'

The attendant looked at me with grateful eyes while the antagonist in this case continued to just stare at me.

I gathered my things and prepared to leave when the individual stopped me.

'Thank you so much,' he said with a smile and continued with folded hands, 'Om Namah Shivay.'

I was caught by surprise. My initial thought of letting him know that he was wrong was replaced by an awkward silence.

'Om Namah Shivay,' I responded slowly with folded hands.

He seemed to preempt my next question.

'My name is Kevin. I am Chinese, and I presume you are Indian,' he said with a smile. 'I love your culture.'

'Oh, that's nice,' I responded.

I introduced myself and asked, 'Where did you learn that greeting?'

'Well, I used to get these images in my dreams right from my childhood,' he replied. 'I realised only recently that these were images of Lord Shiva.'

'That's really intriguing,' I said while actually feeling so.

The next question was even more of a surprise.

'Why is your Lord Shiva blue in colour?'

I was stumped, not only because the question was totally unexpected but because I did not know the answer.

Kevin continued, 'I realised that Lord Shiva is worshipped by Indians.'

This discussion was not up my alley.

'Kevin, I have to leave now,' I said. 'You are an interesting person. Here is my business card. Do come over when you are in that part of town.'

I left the café with 'Om Namah Shivay' still ringing in my ears.

Those were busy days, as I had a rather long list of clients and there was hardly a day when there were no therapy sessions.

## 3

'There is a call for you,' my receptionist, Sandra, said through the intercom.

It was a Saturday afternoon, and I had just finished with a client.

'Please take a message,' I replied and asked out of curiosity, 'Who is the caller?'

Sandra replied, 'He did not reveal his name but asked me to convey the message "Om Namah Shivay".'

'Oh!' I exclaimed and promptly said, 'Please connect me.'

'Om Namah Shivay' were his first words when I answered the phone. 'This is Kevin. I hope you remember me?'

'I do remember you, Kevin,' I responded. 'How are you doing?'

'I am fine,' he replied, 'I want to meet you. When can I come?'

'We can definitely meet,' I assured him and clarified, 'Do you want to talk about religion and culture, or do you have a problem that you want to discuss?'

While they were interesting subjects, I would have very little to contribute.

'I do have a problem,' he said almost on cue.

I suggested a date in the following week, and he agreed.

## 4

There was knock on my door, and he entered. With his lean frame, fair complexion and well-groomed hair, which were nicely complemented by a formal suit and rimless glasses, he did look handsome.

'Om Namah Shivay,' he greeted with a bowed head and folded hands. I stood up and reciprocated.

'Can I touch your feet?' he enquired.

'I am not your guru, Kevin,' I replied, slightly surprised at this strange request. 'In our culture, we usually touch the feet of our guru. Also, in my profession, it is important and an unwritten rule to keep a physical distance from our clients.'

'In that case, can I touch your feet outside?' he persisted.

'Maybe you can do that after the session,' I concluded and beckoned him to sit down.

Once we were both seated, I asked, 'So Kevin, please tell me why you wanted to meet me?'

'I have a problem,' he started and paused.

'You don't look like someone who has a problem,' I said with a chuckle to make him feel more comfortable.

'I am fascinated by my wife,' he continued as if he had not heard me.

'That's lovely. I suppose you have a wonderful relationship with her.'

He responded, 'No, I don't have a relationship. She is no more with me.'

'Oh!' I exclaimed. Are you divorced?'

He hesitated and then whispered, 'She has left me. I have a girlfriend now.'

'So, you have messed up your relationship with your girlfriend,' I surmised.

Maybe that was too direct for him. He remained silent for some time and without any warning, started sobbing. Tears started flowing almost uncontrollably, and he covered his face with his hands.

'Yes,' he admitted amid his outpouring of emotions.

I waited and allowed him time to get his bearings back.

'Kevin, let's talk about your wife and girlfriend later,' I comforted him. 'Tell me more about yourself.'

He composed himself and began his narration.

'I am born Chinese. My father would visit India for his work during the 1970s. Through him, I learnt that most Indians believe in Shiva. He would get a lot of books with pictures in them. These pictures showed that a blue-coloured human lived in Himalayas.'

He closed his eyes and after a few minutes of silence, spoke again. 'Now, whenever I close my eyes and take a deep breath, the pictures of all the animals, all mantras, all the stars fill my head. There is a beautiful waterfall, lake, clear sky, grass field. I can see animals drinking water from the river. There is a bright light with touch of blue running across. Shiva's image is very strong in my head and I keep hearing his mantra, Om Namah Shiva Shiva Shiva.'

He seemed to be besotted by Lord Shiva.

'I have read a lot about Shiva, and it got me interested in spirituality. I read a lot of spiritual books and it makes me happy.'

I waited for him to continue, but he stayed still with his eyes closed.

'How long have you been in Singapore?' I interjected his silence.

He snapped out of his thoughts. 'My parents came here the year I was born. I am here since then.'

'What about your education?' I asked.

'After achieving my A levels, I realised that I was interested in engineering,' he said with a smile. 'I enrolled for an engineering course and now I am a computer engineer.'

'That's wonderful,' I said, nodding my head in appreciation. He was well educated and from a decent family background.

'I was drafted into the National Service, which is a statutory requirement for all male Singaporean citizens. After that, I had to serve two years in the Singapore Armed Forces. I then joined a multinational consulting firm. The job was very good. High profile. Well paying. I travelled to many countries and was doing well. A few years ago, I left the job and started my own company.'

He paused for a moment and continued, 'The company is not doing too well now, but we will turn it around,' he said, trying to put up a brave front.

'Thanks for sharing these details,' I acknowledged.

Now that he was more in control of himself, I went back to where we had left off.

'You were telling me about your girlfriend. What's her name?'

'Vivian,' he said.

'Is she from Singapore?' I asked.

'She is Chinese. She works here.'

'Describe your relationship with her,' I said.

He thought about it, and when he started speaking, his voice was louder. 'She gets hysterical. My logical side tells me that something must be wrong with her. Her physical needs are satisfied.'

I could see his mood changing, and he seemed agitated. 'I cannot stand her rejections. How can she do this to me?'

'What makes you think she is rejecting you?' I enquired.

'Last Friday, I had a huge argument with her. I left home and started walking … to nowhere. I stopped at a street food joint and had dinner. It started raining, but I continued to walk. I realised that I had used some strong words, so I called her to apologise. But she refused to accept my apology. She kept saying that she is upset.'

As he was narrating, I could see his agitation levels increasing.

'Goddammit,' he screamed. 'How can she do that? We had another argument before she slammed the phone. I felt like throwing myself in front of the traffic and killing myself.' He paused and then continued more calmly, 'I reached home late in the evening and she was not at home. I even prepared food for her and went to sleep. The next day, everything was back to normal. I don't feel like coming home anymore.'

'What do you like about her?' I asked, wanting him to share the other side.

His gaze shifted downward, and his eyes suggested that he was digging into his memory bank. I could see his face slowly light up as the more pleasant memories took centre stage.

'She is beautiful,' he said.

'Long hair …

'Great body …

'Soft breasts …

'She is very caring …

'We love each other …'

He closed his eyes and seemed to drift away into his own world.

'Her skin is so soft. I like to run my hands over every part of her body. I could do that for the entire day.'

His expressions suggested that he was fully in the moment that he was describing.

'As I fondle her soft breasts, I can feel her nipples harden. It's like holding a ball of snow. I turn her around as I kiss every part of her tender frame. Her buttocks are so inviting that I cannot resist caressing them. As I become one with her, I am in a valley of flowers with every petal leaving its fragrance,' he reminisced.

It was obvious that his attraction was very physical. I remained unflustered by the graphic details. I watched him as he continued, 'I can never get enough of her. I dream of her even at work.'

His eyes seemed to sparkle with every word as if he was visualising every moment being spoken. For me, something did not feel right. If she was so good, then why the hatred? I looked at my watch. It was getting close to an hour since we had started. I slowly let him come back to his present.

'Kevin, you have shared some details today, but I would like to know more,' I said. 'What would be a good day of the week for you?'

'I would prefer a Saturday, which is not a busy day for me.'

We agreed to meet the following Saturday.

# 5

The person I saw the following Saturday was very different from the Kevin of the previous session. In fact, he was more like the irritable person who had forced me to get up from the sofa at the café.

There was no 'Om Namah Shivay' when he entered. For that matter, there was no greeting at all. His face was red, and his eyes were flaring. He went straight to the chair and looked at me as if to say, 'Get on with it.'

As a therapist, I am used to seeing my clients in a different mood every time they come for a session. It is a reflection of their inability to handle situations which, over some time, are causing some serious challenges in their life or those of others. My first response is always to listen. Listen to what they have to say, listen to their body language, listen to their expressions. It is a proven fact that, more than what people say, it is their nonverbals which reveal a lot about them.

Kevin's nonverbals were screaming anger, confusion, and an inability to control situations; more importantly, they were crying for help.

I did not speak for some time, letting him continue his internal conversations. When his breathing seemed to come back to normal and his demeanour seemed calmer, I initiated the conversation.

'Om Namah Shivay!' I said with a smile.

'Om Namah Shivay,' he responded and managed a sheepish grin, probably realising that he had not greeted me until that point.

'You want to tell me something, Kevin?' It was a rhetorical question. As if waiting for the cue, Kevin jumped in.

'Yesterday, I had gone out for lunch. Vivian asked where I had gone for lunch. I did not want to tell her. Why should I have to tell everything to her?' He looked at me, probably seeking my approval. I did not give any. Seeing no reaction, he continued, 'She goes for Novena every Saturday. Before leaving, she demanded to know with whom I had gone for lunch. The more she demanded, the more I refused to tell her. Why should I? I will not allow her to control my life.'

His breathing was again becoming heavy as he recollected the conversation with his girlfriend.

'She took my keys and left my place. She kept insisting I must tell her. I was so angry that I broke a few plates while washing them. When she came back home, I controlled my anger. Slowly she started to calm down. I went out for dinner, came back, and showered. I wanted sex, but she told me to watch a TV show. I got really angry. This morning, when I was ready to come here, she snatched my keys and did not allow me to leave the house. I pushed her away. She started throwing tantrums, and when she is in this mood, she can be nasty. I just left the house and came here.'

He was fuming now. This also explained his state of mind when he had walked in. I maintained my silence. I could see his anger slowly turn to helplessness as some tears started making their appearance. He seemed morose now as he verbalised his thoughts.

'I was very disappointed,' he murmured amidst the sniffs. 'I feel like giving up on everything. I ask her, do you want to run away from this relationship? She says I will never let you go. I felt upset, disappointed. She is worse than my mother.'

After some thought, he continued, 'I want to run away from all this, but I am still worried about her. I am tired of relationships. I am tired of her questions. I am tired of her suspicious nature. I am tired of her anxiety attacks. If she is normal, I will enjoy her company.'

I came in at this point. 'Kevin, have you ever considered the fact that she cares for you? Maybe she only wants to have a conversation with you. Hence, she is asking where you went for lunch.'

His gaze shifted downward, and it stayed there for what seemed an eternity. 'She does care for me. She does. Yes, she cares for me. Even when she is away at her job, she calls up to enquire about me.'

As if he had remembered something, he said, 'She makes lovely soups,' and the hint of a smile finally made its appearance on his lips.

The smile lasted only for a second before he became pensive again.

'She was not like this. She would understand when I would want to have a conversation and when I would like to be quiet.

When she would come home after a long flight, I would also make food for her.'

And with a smile, he added, 'She loves chicken.'

'Where does she work?' I enquired since we had not discussed that before.

He remained silent seemingly, lost in his own world.

I repeated the question.

'She is an air hostess with Singapore Airlines,' he said in a husky voice. 'She looks so heavenly in uniform. Her buttocks are so inviting that I want to hold them.'

A normal person would have cringed with his constant references to the female anatomy, but as a therapist, I understand that every word spoken by the client tells something about his personality and mindset. Kevin had a craving for physical intimacy.

'I would tell her to wear the uniform in bed and just seeing her lying there for me, all soft and tender, would fill me with ecstasy.'

It was now getting embarrassing even for me, and I intervened.

'She may be travelling a lot,' I said.

He looked up. 'She is away for four days of the week, but I am fine with that, as that's her job.'

Until now, all his narrations had been all about himself—what he wants and is getting or otherwise. This was probably the first time he was looking at things from the perspective of others.

I said, 'From what you are saying, Kevin, your girlfriend does care for you. What is bothering you is her wanting to know more details about what you are doing, which you feel is her controlling behaviour.'

He nodded, and I continued.

'How would it feel if you stopped reacting to it? You said she loves you. When she does ask you where you had lunch and with whom, do not react. Just answer her. She may ask you ten times. Answer her ten times. Would that be possible?'

His reaction suggested that he was not convinced. In fact, I could sense a hint of irritation.

'She has these panic attacks. She wants to know everything. I feel suffocated.' He grimaced.

'Kevin, you shared your dreams about Shiva. You said that you read a lot of spiritual books. What would those books tell you to do in this situation?' I asked, wanting him to seek some answers from within himself.

That made him think, and he said, 'When I am really depressed, I practise meditation. I go to a centre where they teach "humming by throat" meditation. After the meditation, I feel so much better.'

That was rather unexpected coming from someone who needed a lot of it, but it was very useful information which I could use to help him. I had heard about 'humming by throat' but did not know enough. I made a note to do some reading on it.

With the clock showing that the session was nearing its completion, I proceeded to share a summary.

'Kevin, I understand that you have a hot and cold relationship with your girlfriend. You said that she cares for you, but sometimes she becomes very controlling, and then you don't like all the questions that she keeps asking. You feel that she was not like this before and that she would understand your needs better. Something has changed, and you don't know what.'

I moved on to some suggestions.

'Kevin, you understand spirituality, and hence, you will also know that the answer to a lot of our problems lies within us. You may expect your girlfriend to change and be the person she was before, but that is not in your control. What is in your control is how you react in situations which make your angry, irritable, and frustrated. Although it may not be easy, try doing what I said before. Just answer her questions as many times as she asks them. Let her think she is controlling you. You know that you are doing it to avoid her tantrums and make you calmer.'

He was nodding his head and listening intently.

'Kevin, it's never about anyone else. It is always about you and what you can control. Let's meet on Saturday of next week, and you can share how you managed to do it.'

Kevin nodded again but said nothing. He may still not be convinced, but I wanted to plant a seed in his head which I would slowly nurture and grow in future sessions.

That night, I went to the internet and did some reading on 'humming meditation'.

> Humming is a technique designed to open us to trust, to bring us into our inner sanctuary of peace and serenity. It has ancient roots in Tibetan Buddhist techniques. As we hum, we generate our own energy to heal and Center ourselves. Humming brings us straight down from the head and into the body, keeping us alert yet relaxed. The sounds resonating throughout the body/mind have a soothing, calming effect. It is particularly good for healing the heart on both the emotional and physical levels, for releasing emotional distress, and for bringing us to a balanced state of deeply centred well-being. It is also helpful for anyone who suffers from throat, bronchial, lung, or chest problems

or who has communication difficulties, and it
is ideal for singers or speakers or anyone who
wants to become a singer or speaker.

# 6

Come Saturday, Sandra informed me that Kevin had called
and rescheduled his appointment from that afternoon to the
Tuesday of the following week.

With no other appointments scheduled on that day, I took a
break on Saturday and spent the day at the One⁰15 Marina club,
where I am a member. I did some swimming in their infinity
swimming pool and indulged myself with a soothing massage at
the spa centre, leaving a more refreshed version of myself. A little
pampering from time to time is good for the mind and body.

Another version of Kevin walked into my clinic on Tuesday.
From the time he stepped in, he was fidgety, and his expressions
suggested that he was lost. After the usual greetings, I asked him
the reason for rescheduling the session.

'I had to travel to Turkey on business,' he explained. 'I
am trying to set up a new partnership to get entry into the
European market.'

'Was the trip successful?' I enquired.

'Uh … the trip? Oh yes, I had some initial discussions, but
nothing is finalised yet,' he said with some hesitation.

'What's the matter?' I asked, sensing his uneasiness.

After some thought, he said, 'I met a girl there. She was the
receptionist at the company I was visiting. She was beautiful. She
had long hair and lovely eyes. I asked her out, and she agreed.
One thing led to another, and we spent the night together. I
don't feel good about it.' His eyes showed a tinge of remorse.

'And why is that?' I asked.

'This is all because of Vivian,' he suddenly screamed. 'If she had not denied sex, I would never have done this.'

'So, you blame your act on her?' I asked in a tone which gave more than a hint of my response.

'We would have sex two to three times every night,' he revealed. 'She would scream loudly whenever I entered her from behind. She did not like it, but she did it anyway. Why does she have to deny it now?'

He had ventured into the physical aspects of his relationship again.

'What do you think?' I probed.

His response was not an answer to the question.

'She was so different earlier. She would do everything I wanted her to do.' He closed his eyes as he recollected the moments he was describing, 'Even after a long flight, she would never complain of any tiredness. We would lie in bed without any clothes, her buttocks pressing against my penis as I caressed her soft breasts. Now, after a few hours of work, she gets a headache. If I ask her anything, she gets hysterical.'

This was getting even more gross, but I decided to ignore the description and focus on the essence of what he was saying.

'Maybe she is having some genuine health problem,' I countered.

'All of you are the same,' he screamed. 'You only blame me. I cannot trust anyone. Even in my past life, I was betrayed. My hands were cut off, and I was beheaded.'

*Past life!* I thought. This was different but not entirely surprising given his spiritual leanings. I decided to play along.

'Who has betrayed you?' I asked.

He stared at me and continued, 'She put a tape recorder in the office and recorded my laughter. That was after reading my friend's email, but she thought I was having an affair with another girl in the office. I even asked her to check with car park security. She did all this because she wanted the property and business. I would have given her all of it anyway.

'Vivian did that?' I sought clarification.

'No, Rachel,' he responded.

'Who is Rachel?' I asked.

'My wife,' he said as if it was so obvious.

I was getting confused here. Whom was he talking about?

'So, Rachel betrayed you?' I asked.

He seemed unsure of his response. His thoughts seemed to be all messed up.

'Vivian is an air hostess?' I asked, seeking another clarification.

'No!' was his nonchalant response. 'Rachel is an air hostess.'

My thoughts were a loud *What?* but my verbal response was 'OK.'

'Your ex-wife, right?' I quizzed.

'She was so beautiful. I fell in love with her the moment I saw her in London. We had such a wonderful time.'

'Why did you get separated?' I probed this new piece of information.

His uneasiness increased, and his body started twitching.

'I wanted to give her a surprise. I went to her office, but it was locked from inside. I knocked on the door. She took almost fifteen minutes to open the door. When I went in, he was there. I was very angry but did not lose my control.'

'Who was there?' I interrupted.

'Mark' was his simple response.

'And who is Mark?' I asked.

'He is the office manager,' he said.

'Why were you angry?'

'Why did they have to lock the door?' he screamed in response. 'I did not confront her, but after some days, I found some letter in her cupboard which made it very clear that she was having an affair.'

He broke down.

'Why did she betray me?' he sobbed.

'Where is she now?' I asked.

'Um ... she is here,' he replied in an uncertain tone.

'In Singapore?' I asked.

'Um ...' he replied.

I had a strong lead now which could be explored, but there was still a lot of confusion that needed to be cleared.

'After she left, Vivian came into your life ... right?' I checked.

'Vivian is my girlfriend,' he said emphatically.

'And you love her?' I enquired.

'Yes' was his monosyllabic response.

I was perplexed now. All this while, I was under the impression that he did love his girlfriend but they were having a lot of issues lately, which was why he was coming to me. His latest statement suggested otherwise, and the separation from his wife seemed to be the real cause. Nothing was adding up.

Without being judgmental, I proceeded to know more about his girlfriend, Vivian.

'For how long you have known Vivian?' I asked.

'More than a year now,' he replied.

'How did you meet her?'

His fidgeting continued, and it was difficult to ascertain whether he was uncomfortable or uncertain with my line of questioning. I decided to continue.

'When did you meet her for the first time?' I asked.

'She is my neighbour,' he finally responded. 'She took care of me when I was not well. She would bring me food to eat and comfort me. She is beautiful. Long hair, big breasts …'

I pretended to listen as he described her anatomy in minute detail.

'One night, she came home with a cake. It was my birthday. We kept talking until very late. I had not had sex for many days and wanted it desperately. We were on the couch, and I leaned forward and kissed her.'

He adjusted his position on the chair as he continued speaking.

'She did not push me away. I felt her soft lips for the first time. I gently ran my fingers through her hair and pulled her closer to me. She began to respond slowly. Her hands came around my back, and I could feel her body stiffening. I slowly let my hands move down her back and lifted her loose top. As I touched the skin of her back, I felt a tingling sensation all over. I wanted her so much. I slowly unhooked her bra and let it fall. She had the biggest breasts of all the women I had been with. I caressed them gently, and she moaned. I kissed the dark nipples and started biting them gently. She was enjoying this as her cries of ecstasy became louder. I could wait no longer. I unbuttoned her pants and pulled them down. I almost tore my shirt and pulled down my pants. I so wanted her. As I pulled her towards me, she was all hot, and the tiny hairs on her hands were all standing up. I turned her around and entered her from behind. She gave a loud groan and pulled away. She turned to face me and pulled me down over her. I kept riding every wave of ecstasy until it was done. I can still feel the smooth skin, the softness of her breasts, and the smell of her body.'

Finally, he fell silent. He lay there with his eyes closed, probably as spent as he had been at the end of the moment he had just described.

He had shared the intimate details of that encounter so vividly that I was also lost for words. I could only stare at him. As if all this was not enough, he suddenly found his voice again.

'She was wonderful in bed. We would have sex two to three times a night.'

I had to intervene now before he went into more details. Sex seemed to play a very important role in all his relationships.

'What changed?' I asked.

'What?' he responded

'I mean, if the two of you were getting along so well, I wonder why you would have the frequent fights could be that you have been describing?'

'What fights?' he asked.

'You have been telling about your fights with your girlfriend. That she questions you and probably controls you,' I reminded him.

He stared at me for a few seconds, and then the twitching and fidgeting increased. He kept shaking his head and murmured something, probably in Chinese.

'I don't know,' he muttered.

Kevin was in a different frame of mind, and there was no point in taking the discussion further when it was difficult to verify the veracity of his statements.

I reiterated the need to restrain himself when faced with a barrage of questions, although I was not sure how much of it was comprehended.

# 7

In my twenty years of practice, I had never encountered an incident where I had to get involved with my client beyond the planned sessions. With experience, I had devised various therapies to create a better impact for my clients, and accordingly, I would engage with them outside the clinic. However, these would be strictly restricted to the objective of the therapy.

This was about to change.

The distant sound of my mobile phone's ring tone woke me up. Before I could gather my wits, the ringing stopped. I looked at the clock next to my bed. It was 11:21 p.m. Just as I was trying to figure out whether it was dream, the phone rang again.

It was an unknown number.

'Am I speaking to Dr Preeti Pandit?' the voice at the other end said.

'Yes,' I answered hesitantly.

'I am Officer James Carter from the local police centre,' the person said.

Getting a call from the police—and at this time of the night—is the last thing I would have expected.

'Do you know a Mr Kevin Liu?' the officer asked.

'Yes, Officer,' I replied slowly.

'May I know in what relation do you know him?' the officer asked.

'I am his psychotherapist. He is my client,' I answered, not sure where this was leading.

'I request that you come to the police station. Mr Kevin is here, and he needs you. I am sending a squad car to pick you up,' he said.

'Why does he need me, Officer?' I asked.

'Please come. We will explain. Thank you,' he said bluntly and hung up.

I woke up Pankaj and tried explaining the situation to him. He seemed very reluctant to let me go to the police station at that hour, but I insisted.

'Hello, Officer,' I said when I reached Officer James Carter's desk. 'I am Dr Preeti Pandit.'

'Thank you for coming, Doctor,' he said. 'Please sit down.'

'We have brought Mr Kevin Liu and his girlfriend Vivian Chang. One Mr John Barnes has filed a complaint against them.'

'Oh!' I muttered.

'Eyewitnesses say that Ms Vivian Chang was seen to be screaming in the middle of the street. Mr Kevin Liu was trying to calm her down, but they got into a quarrel instead. They were very loud. The lady started throwing stones at the man, and one of them happened to hit a cab driver, who has filed the complaint.'

'Oh!' I grimaced.

The officer continued, 'Kevin has given a statement that he is undergoing therapy with you. Is that right?'

'Yes, Officer,' I replied.

He wrote something in his book and continued, 'He has also stated that during his sessions, he has mentioned that his girlfriend is suffering from severe depression and is prone to panic attacks. Is that right?' he asked.

'Yes, Officer,' I replied.

'Can I see your identity proof, Doctor?' he asked.

Having verified my identity, the officer stated, 'Based on your evidence, we are not taking any further action against Mr Kevin Liu and Miss Vivian Chang on health grounds. Are you willing to sign on this undertaking?' he asked.

Not having an option, I obliged.

Once the formalities were done, the officer first apologised, thanked me for my time, and instructed a junior officer to drop me back home.

I made a mental note to call Kevin first thing in the morning.

## 8

Even before I did, I received a call from Kevin early the next day.

'I am so sorry to get you involved in all this,' he started with an apology.

'I did my duty Kevin,' I said, 'although I was not too happy at having to visit the police station in the middle of the night.'

'When we were taken to the police station, you were the first person who came to my mind. You are always so calm and assured. Also, I thought that giving a medical reason for whatever happened was the best way to avoid getting charged.'

It was a smart move, but I did not want to admit it.

'Can I come and meet you on Saturday?' he asked.

'I would like to meet you sooner,' I said. He explained, 'I am travelling to Bangkok for some work tonight and will be back only by Friday. Hence, I am requesting for an appointment on Saturday.'

'In that case, let's meet at 2 p.m. on Saturday,' I said and hung up.

## 9

I had my calendar planned for Saturday and reached the clinic early. Sandra greeted me with a warm smile.

'Good morning, ma'am,' she said.

'Good morning, dear,' I responded. 'How are you doing today?'

'All is well ma'am,' she replied. 'There is a message for you from Mr Kevin.'

'What is it?' I asked, almost in anticipation of something unexpected.

She read from her notes: 'He called a few minutes ago and said that he had to extend his stay in Bangkok and hence will not be able to come for the session today. He has requested for an appointment next week, on any day, based on your schedules. He is ready to adjust his work accordingly.'

I was peeved at these last-minute changes. I am a stickler for commitments, and the lack of it in others is the one thing which irks me.

'He asked me to convey his sincere apologies and will be calling in an hour to know your response,' she added and put the notepad down.

'Could you please check my calendar and suggest a good time, Sandra?' I requested.

'I have already done that, ma'am. Tuesday and Wednesday afternoons are free. Shall I pencil him in for Tuesday?' she asked with a smile of satisfaction.

'Yes, please do that,' I confirmed and acknowledged her presence of mind.

I thought, *This is the second time Kevin is rescheduling his appointments. He seems to be all over the place with his life.*

Tuesday came, and another version of Kevin walked into my clinic. He seemed happy, and a smile lit his face. He bowed and greeted me and almost bounced into his chair. He seemed very unlike any of his earlier versions.

'Let me first apologise to you for the unfortunate incident,' he started almost immediately.

The police station incident seemed a distant memory due to the time that had elapsed, but I acknowledged his apology with a nod of my head.

I gave a candid summary: 'Kevin, we have met three times before, and you have shared a lot of details about yourself; your girlfriend, Vivian; and your ex-wife, Rachel. However, all the details have been in bits and pieces, and I am not able to join them together. If you are really looking at me for help, you need to provide me with all the details that you can possibly remember and then be disciplined in doing what we agree in the session.'

'Dr Pandit, I agree that I have not been disciplined, but I have been honest. I don't know why, but from the time I met you, I have felt that you are the person who can help me. You are so warm and caring. Your voice has a soothing effect on me, and I feel so good when I am with you,' he confessed. 'I want a better life and need your help to achieve it.'

'Have you visited any other therapist or doctor?' I asked.

'Yes, I have taken treatment for depression from Dr Chew Choon Seng, a psychiatrist. That was about six months ago. I still take the medications he has prescribed,' he shared.

'Do you still visit him?' I asked.

He replied, 'I have not gone to him for many months now.'

I asked him to get the prescription when we meet next, and he agreed.

'Kevin, tell me what happened that night?' I asked.

He thought for a moment and said, 'When I reached home from work, Vivian began questioning me as she always does. She wanted to know why I have to travel so much. I had just returned from Turkey so that was probably the trigger. I was tired and did not want to talk to her. But she kept insisting. She accused me of having an affair and not paying any attention to her. She started throwing things in the house. I had to slap her to calm her down, but she got even more hysterical. She started abusing me and when I shouted back, she left the house. She started screaming from the street, so I had to go down. I requested her to calm down and come back into the house, but she refused. I got very angry and threatened to kill her. She picked up some stones and threw at me. Unfortunately, they hit a passing cab. The cab driver filed a complaint and we had to present ourselves.'

He looked at me 'She is losing it. Earlier, she used to get panic attacks once a week but lately it has become a daily affair. I am sick and tired of this nonsense.'

He was getting agitated again.

'Every day I come home; it is the same story. She will ask me why I was late, with whom I had lunch, why am I smelling differently. Am I only here to answer her questions?' he bellowed

I intervened 'Kevin, is she undergoing treatment with someone?'

'No ... I don't think so,' he confessed after some thought.

'Can you bring her here? I would like to meet her,' I asked.

'Here ...!' He hesitated. 'If she meets you, she is going to start suspecting something between us.'

'Why would that happen? Let's give it a try,' I suggested.

He was not too sure.

'Let me think about it,' he said as if trying to change the topic.

'I think she needs help,' I said in an assertive tone, wanting to drive home a point. 'There must be a reason for the panic attacks, and it is important we identify them since it is also having a big impact on your life. Don't you want to see her come back to normal? You say that she has taken care of you during your bad times. Shouldn't you do something to help her in her difficult time?'

His gaze shifted downwards, and he was silent. I could see the tears making their appearance, which suggested that my words were having an impact.

'You are right. I should take care of her. She has been so nice to me,' he confessed.

'All this while, I have been so selfish. I have only bothered about myself. What must she be going through?' He clenched his fists and banged it on the handle of the chair. 'How can I be so irresponsible? Everyone makes a mistake. I should have given her a chance. I could have prevented the divorce.'

It was like a bolt that hit me. This seemed a case of schizophrenia.

All this while, I have been trying to understand the problem, and here it was, staring at me.

'You don't have to be so severe on yourself, Kevin,' I said, now even more curious to know his line of thought.

He looked up at me with pangs of guilt in his eyes still not reassured by my words.

'I don't think so. I should blame myself for the divorce.' He was sobbing uncontrollably now. 'If I was more understanding and less selfish, we could still be together. Career is important for some people. How can I deny her that? If she had the baby at that time, it may have affected her career. She was right in going through with the abortion.'

He had started speaking about something very different, but it was clear that he was talking about Rachel.

'Did she have an abortion?' I asked.

'Yes, we had a huge argument, and I gave her a choice. Either she goes through with the abortion or we get divorced,' he said between the flood of tears.

'And what did she choose?' I asked.

His voice grew louder. 'She chose her career. That was more important for her. So typical of her to do that.' The tears were giving way to anger again. 'It's always about her. Even when I am tired and don't want to talk about anything, she has to ask those hundred questions.'

He was switching between personalities again. His thoughts were getting all messed up. He was doing this so often, leaving himself with a confused set of emotions.

I leaned forward and looked him in the eye.

'Kevin, how committed are you to improve your life?' I asked.

He was slightly taken aback but responded, 'That's the only thing I want now.'

'Kevin, if you are indeed committed, please listen to me. This is what I want you to do,' I said sternly. 'From tomorrow, you will attend humming by throat meditation everyday. Practise the same every morning when you wake up. During the day, you are going to answer every question that Vivian asks you whether you are tired or not. And you are not going to show any emotion while doing that. Can you do that?'

'I will attend the meditation course daily,' he said but added cautiously, 'but the other thing is difficult.'

'Change is always difficult, Kevin, and there is no change if it is not difficult. If you want your life to change, you have to do this,' I said strongly.

'OK,' he said, but the conviction was not there.

I looked him in the eye and continued strongly, 'Kevin, we would be wasting each other's time if you are only going to come here and tell me your story. If it was easy to change things, you would have already done that by now. You decided to take my help because you felt you needed someone else to show you the way. I am showing you the way now. But it is you who have to walk that path.'

This time, his response was better. 'I understand, Dr Pandit. I want a better life, and I will do what is necessary.'

'It's time for action now. Let me know on Saturday.'

## 10

Another Saturday dawned, and another message from Kevin. This time, it was an apology in advance for his late arrival.

'Om Namah Shivay,' he said, trying to catch his breath, suggesting that he had rushed to the session from wherever he had been in the morning.

'Om Namah Shivay!' I greeted him and gave him a look. The silence spoke.

'I sincerely apologise for the inconvenience again,' he pleaded. 'I had to be in Bangkok again this week, and my flight got delayed.'

'Kevin, making a mistake is part of being human,' I explained. 'However, you cannot make the same mistake more than once, because the next time you do it, it's not a mistake anymore. It's a choice. Be careful of the choices you make in life.'

His expression suggested that my point had hit where it hurts most.

'I was not like this,' he moaned. 'I have always wanted things to happen in a structured manner. There are too many things happening in my life.'

'Kevin, have you been attending the meditation sessions?' I asked.

'Yes, Dr Pandit, except when I am away in Bangkok,' he replied.

'Have you been listening to Vivian more and trying to respond to her questions positively?' I asked.

He stammered, 'Well … I am trying … but it's difficult.'

I wanted to ensure that he was doing what we had agreed to do during our earlier sessions.

'Kevin, please have a glass of water and relax,' I instructed.

Kevin did as told and took a comfortable position on the therapy chair.

I leaned forward on my chair and looked straight in his eyes.

'Kevin, I want you feel relaxed. I will be giving you some instructions now. I want you to follow them without thinking too much into it. Do it with sincerity, and trust your subconscious mind to help you in this process,' I explained to him calmly. I continued in a soft tone, 'Please close your eyes now and concentrate on your breath. Relax every part of your body. Focus on your breath as you inhale and exhale.' I let him stay there for a few minutes.

'I invite you to focus your mind on your ex-wife, Rachel. Let your thoughts wander into the far corners of your mind, and get all the memories associated with her. All the moments you have sent with her. All your thoughts about her.'

I could see the muscles of his face and his fingers twitching. His expressions changed every few seconds, which suggested that his life events playing in his head.

'She is so beautiful. So petite. I love the way her long hair blows in the breeze and the way she pushes the curls away from her face …'

'Kevin, I invite you to a time before your wedding. Recollect the moments spent with Rachel. Let it play in slow motion. Experience every emotion that you are feeling.'

I let him be with Rachel for some time. A gentle smile dotted his face. 'She makes me feel so nice about myself. Even when I am agitated, she has a calm way of dealing with me ...'

'Kevin, I want you to now recollect all the moments which led to your marriage with her. Experience your feelings for her. Request your subconscious mind to tell you the reasons why you married her.'

I waited and watched his heavy breathing to understand that he was still connected with his past. 'I knew she was the one for me. No one had filled my moments with so much happiness. Life was so beautiful when I was with her ...'

Considering the emphasis he had been placing physical intimacy, I let him live some of those moments as well.

'Kevin, I want you to be with Rachel and bring alive the moments you spent with her in bed. Experience those intimate moments the two of you shared.'

His expressions suggested that he was really into it now. 'I am running my fingers gently over her smooth body. I kiss her soft breasts and gently press them. She guides my hand between her legs and moans softly when I use my fingers to arouse her. She lets me do what I want to ...'

'I now invite you to be a part of your wedding. Watch the event as it unfolds before you as if you are watching a movie. Increase the volume, brighten the picture, increase the contrast of the picture you are seeing. You are in control, Kevin.'

His facial muscles were telling me that he was going through a flood of emotions. 'We are in the church, and the choir is playing in the background. I lift her veil and see her lovely eyes. We kiss as husband and wife and the whole world is showering their love ...'

'Please continue, Kevin. What else do you see?' I ask.

'Life is wonderful. I decide to start my own business. I have opened my new office. I am giving the power of attorney of my new business to her. We are so happy.'

I softly intervene.

'I now invite you to zoom into the events after your marriage. As you see these events playing in front of you, try to identify the events which affected your relationship.'

He continued after a pause.

'Rachel is pregnant. I am so happy. I feel on top of the world. And ... and ...'

He stopped, and his entire body started twitching. He had recollected something really discomforting.

I asked, 'Kevin, tell me what you see?'

'She is telling me that she wants to abort the baby. I can't believe it. She says it will not be good for her career. I try to convince her. I plead with her. After some days, she tells me that she has aborted the baby. She killed my baby. How could she do that?'

He started sobbing uncontrollably. The tears were an indication of all the pent-up emotions inside him which were not finding a right channel to come out. I let him be.

I could see that he is in great discomfort, but the therapy had helped him reach a state which was necessary to liberate him. I had to continue.

'Go back to the moment when she tells you about the abortion. Now, move on from there. What is happening now?' I urged gently.

After a moment of silence, he continued, 'She has called me to the office. Her manager is there with her. She tells me ...'

And he stopped.

'What is she telling you, Kevin? Increase the volume,' I urge softly.

He continues slowly, 'She tells me that it is all over. She tells me that she has taken over the company. She tells me that she wants a divorce and asks me to sign the divorce papers. If I don't sign, she will report to the police that I have illegally started this business while still being employed. She is laughing now. He is also laughing. I am devastated. I am pleading with her … and … and … I am signing the divorce papers.'

He bursts into tears again. The strain of going back in time, reliving the moments, and experiencing the variety of emotions that he described would have drained him.

'Kevin, I want you to come back to the present and take control of yourself,' I said softly when the outburst ceased.

He wiped the tears, took a few sips of water, and looked at me. His face was puffed with all the crying. His eyes were red and hair dishevelled. He seemed completely disoriented.

One thing remained.

I asked 'Kevin, based on what you experienced just now, are there any realisations?'

He took a while to speak.

'I truly loved Rachel. I trusted her with everything—my life, my business, my money—and she took it all away,' he shared as his voice choked.

'What could you have done about the situation, Kevin?' I asked.

'Maybe, I shouldn't have given her the power of attorney,' he thought aloud.

'Would that have changed anything?' I probed.

'Maybe … I would probably still have my business … and my money,' he murmured.

'What about the love that you shared? What about that?' I probed further.

'No, I don't think so. Once the trust is gone, there can be no love,' he pondered.

*Bullseye*, I thought.

'What does this tell you?' I threw the final salvo.

He was deep in thought.

'I have been holding onto something which was never there. She never loved me. She married me for my money,' he said in anger.

I intervened to balance his thoughts. 'It may not be that bad. The deep love that you shared with her before your marriage and for many months after marriage must have been real. No one can pretend to love you for so long. The lure of money, power, attraction to her manager, or a combination of these could have become more important for her than the love for you. However, what is important is your realisation that you were not to blame for whatever happened and that you have to let go.'

He thought about it and said in a more assured tone, 'I agree, Dr Pandit.'

## 11

For the next few weeks, the object of my therapy was Rachel and his love for her. Considering the intensity of his love for her, it was going to take some time before he would come around to accept the reality of the situation with her.

During these weeks, I was happy to see Kevin giving his full commitment to the therapy. He was regular at the meditation sessions, although his bittersweet relationship with Vivian continued. That was my next objective anyway. What irked me, however, was his frequent requests for change of schedule or his coming late for the sessions. In most cases, the reason would be his trips to Bangkok. I decided to do something about it.

'How is business?' I asked Kevin when we started the session.

As was now the practice, Kevin was late.

'It's looking good,' he said with a smile. 'The new year looks like a year full of hope.'

'Are you setting up something in Bangkok?' I asked.

It seemed to catch him off guard, and he started searching for the right response.

He gave a huge sigh and leaned forward. 'I have been meaning to talk to you about this,' he said.

'Go on,' I said calmly.

'I am seeing someone in Bangkok,' he said without looking me in the eye.

'Tell me more,' I said without conveying any emotions.

After some hesitation, he started talking.

'Her name is Rose. I met her a few months ago at a party. She has long hair and lovely eyes. I liked her bubbliness. After the party, we hooked up. I thought it was the end of it, but she called me after a few days saying that she was completely into me. I was having these fights with Vivian and felt so happy with Rose. So, I visited her again in Bangkok. We had sex many times. I could not resist myself, and now I am forced to travel to Bangkok every week.'

'So, you travel to Bangkok only to meet Rose?' I asked.

He hesitated and then admitted, 'Yes.'

I continued to just look at him, which probably made him defensive.

'You cannot blame me, Dr Pandit. I have been so happy over the past few weeks.'

I must agree that he had seemed happier during the recent sessions.

'You know what is so good about her? She wants me. She does not ask me any questions. We just talk and have sex. She is petite. Her breasts are so soft, and she lets me do it the way I want to.'

'Just like Rachel?' I interrupted.

'Ah!' he uttered as he tried to make sense of my question.

I had my answer.

He continued, 'We have sex before I catch the flight, and hence, I have missed some of my flights. Sometimes, she insists I stay back for the weekend as well.'

He looked at me sheepishly. I remained silent and kept looking at him without showing any emotion.

'I know I shouldn't be doing this, but it is all because of Vivian,' he remarked.

'Kevin, let's talk about Vivian,' I said. 'You have been doing humming by throat meditation for a few weeks now. You have also managed to let go of Rachel. How is your relationship with Vivian now?'

'I see less of her now,' he admitted. 'Whenever I am at home, I feel that I do not react as much to her nagging.'

'Let's spend some time with Vivian today. Would you want to do that?' I asked.

'Yes,' he answered.

I started the therapy and let his thoughts wander into the past and reach the point where he met Vivian for the first time.

He narrated what he was seeing through his mind's eye: 'I am heartbroken since Rachel left me. I may not have eaten for a couple of days. I am very weak and have collapsed on the stairway of my apartment block. Vivian finds me there and helps me to my apartment. For the next few days, she brings my groceries, cooks food for me, and engages in long conversations with me. She has also lost her parents in an accident recently. She is lonely. I am comforting her.'

He paused as a realisation seemed to dawn upon him.

'She is so good to me. In a few days, I am feeling so much better. I start going back to work. It is my birthday. She gets a cake for me. We have sex for the first time. It is wonderful. She lets me do things to her. We have sex every day, sometimes two or three times.'

At an opportune moment, I intervened.

'Kevin, request your subconscious mind to fast forward to the time when things started to go wrong in your relationship.'

He remained silent as I encouraged him gently to keep trying. I could see some creases appearing on his forehead as he strained his memory and finally started speaking.

'She wants me to call every hour when I am at work. As soon as I come home, she wants me to tell her everything. She gets upset when I have to travel. She checks my phone and asks me why I am getting some messages. I am beginning to feel suffocated. I tell her that she has changed. She is angry and starts shouting. I calm her down. I tell her sorry. She also hugs me and tells me that I should never leave her.'

I wait for him to continue and then slowly urge him.

'Kevin, I want you to imagine having sex with Vivian. How is it different?'

He is calm at first and then starts twitching.

'She has a lovely body, and I crave to hold her big breasts. They are so firm. I kiss her lips gently and move my lips over every part of her, and she starts moaning. She is very loud. As the volcano is about to erupt, I turn her around and want to do things with her. She wants it the other way around. She is guiding me through her body. She is moaning ever so loudly, and we are there.'

I can see him breathing heavily, but I want him to talk more.

'You had wonderful sex with Vivian. Why are you not satisfied?' I asked.

'It was wonderful,' he said, still panting, 'but I wish she would allow me to do it from behind. She would do that earlier but not now.'

I had heard what I wanted to. I let his breathing return to normal.

'Kevin, I want you to think of all the recent interactions with Vivian and narrate them to me.'

It was not too difficult to make him speak since these were incidents from his recent memory.

'She wants to know why my shirt is smelling differently. She accuses me of having an affair. I am convincing her. Again, she starts shouting. I am not able to control her. I go into my room and shut the door. I open the door the next morning, and she has fallen down outside the door. Her body is hot. I take her to a doctor, who tells me she is in depression.'

After some moments of silence, he continues.

'I am confused. My business needs my time. She wants me around all the time. What should I do?'

His entire body is now twitching, which suggests he is very uncomfortable with what is going in his head. I slowly bring him back to the present and help him bring his breathing to normal. When he is back in the present, I ask him to reflect.

'Vivian was so warm and caring initially. I was so happy. We had wonderful sex, but then she got into a state of depression. She started controlling me, which drew me away from her.'

I leaned forward and looked him in the eye.

'Kevin, I want you to really think and answer,' I said. 'When she was warm and caring, whom did she remind you of?'

His eyes suggested that he was searching for an answer.

'When you were having sex with her, she was like ...' I trailed off.

'Rachel!' he replied promptly.

His expression changed to one of bewilderment.

'Holy shit,' he gasped under his breath as the realisation began to dawn upon him. I could sense that he was playing back some of the memories that he had experienced as if to confirm this realisation. 'Oh my God!' he exclaimed as he ran his hands through his hair almost pulling at them.

I felt relieved. I had taken him through a journey in the past and made him relive the bittersweet experiences. There was a high risk involved in this approach, but I realised that was the only way to free him from the web of memories that entangled him.

'She was all good until she was allowing you to do what you wanted to do. When you were having sex with her, what was she not doing?' I asked.

'She would not allow me to take her from behind,' he said.

'Which is how Rachel wanted it,' I added.

'Oh my God,' he gasped. 'That's right.'

'And that's how the girl in Bangkok wants it as well?' I suggested.

The realisation dawned on him like a bolt of lightning.

'You are right,' he muttered.

## 12

During the past few weeks, the therapy has helped Kevin realise that he had to let go of Rachel as she was in the past. He has also realised that the sex with Rachel was a very special part of that relationship and probably what he may be missing more than anything else.

The relationship with Vivian was an outlet for satisfying his sexual urges, and it was always Rachel in bed with him. It worked well until he was able to get what he wanted from Vivian, especially in bed. When Vivian started demanding more from the relationship and wanting her way in bed, he could no longer see Rachel in her. The other sexual escapades in Turkey, Bangkok, and other places were his subconscious search for the sex that he was missing since he split with Rachel.

It had been almost eight months since we had started our sessions. It had been draining for me and most definitely for Kevin. I now wanted him to start living his own life, without my influence. I planned to have that conversation today.

'Why do you want to stop meeting me?' he said when I suggested that we need not meet every week.

I explained, 'As a therapist, my job is to help my clients come out of the hole that they find themselves in. I will do everything necessary to pull them out of the hole. Once they are out, I have to let them live their life, on their own terms. You are at that stage now.'

'This is not fair,' he remarked. 'I am feeling so good about myself. I am beginning to realise that life is beautiful, and now you tell me that we will not have our sessions. This is not fair.'

I smiled and replied in a tongue-in-cheek manner, 'You have been meeting me every week for the past eight months, Kevin. Of course you are going to feel good.'

That elicited laughter from him as well.

'However, I will just not leave you without first ensuring that you have the resources to face the world,' I assured him.

'Oh, that's good,' he said with a relieved smile.

'Have you heard of Vipassana?' I asked.

He was blank.

'No, what's that?' he asked.

'It is one of the oldest forms of Buddhist meditation. It is very difficult, but once you do manage to do it, your life will be transformed,' I explained.

'That's interesting.' He nodded his head.

'Kevin, from the time you first greeted me with an "Om Namah Shivay", I felt that you had spiritual leanings. You have seen the benefits of humming by throat meditation. You have taken a lot of efforts to slowly bring your life back on track. Now is the right time to thoroughly cleanse your being and start a new life.'

His eyes began to sparkle with interest.

'If you are recommending it, it must be good,' he said.

I said, 'I am recommending it because I myself have gone through it. There is a centre in India which is the best in the world. They have a ten-day course, which I attended a couple of years ago. I am a transformed person now.'

'I am doing it. Please help me join the course,' he requested.

Dhamma Giri is one of the world's largest Vipassana meditation centres. It is at Igatpuri in Maharashtra, which is approximately 100 km from Mumbai.

The centre is very strict in implementing the teachings of the Buddha. During the ten days at the centre, you are cut off from the world in every sense of the word. If any person is found to disrespect the norms laid out, he or she is immediately asked to rest the mind in their respective room and is not allowed to leave the ashram's premises for ten days.

I remembered my visit to the centre in 2010. I had no clue about how the Divine had continually guided me and made me enrol for this course. When I reached the centre, my belongings were all taken away. This included all the jewellery I was wearing, my mobile phone, my wallet, and all the money I was carrying. I was left only with the clothes I was wearing, which were also taken away after I donned the simple white outfit that was given to me. I received a room for myself. The room only had a bed and a fan, and this was my abode for the next ten days. I was told that I had to maintain complete silence during the ten days and was not allowed to speak to anyone. I was really scared.

When I entered the dhamma hall the next morning at 4 a.m., it actually felt like heaven. I had never experienced this sense of calm and tranquillity ever. I felt a huge surge of energy in my body, which drained away all my fears. I would spend a large part of the day listening to discourses. When I was back in my room, I would spend time meditating and reflecting on my life and what I have been doing with it. By the seventh day, I felt that my body was not in my control; it seemed some energy outside was operating my mind and body. From the eighth day of meditation, when I would sleep in my room or lie down on my bed, I felt a strange feeling of oneness with the universe.

When I shared some of these details with Kevin, he was all excited.

The only problem was that the courses are booked many months in advance. The next day, I called Mr Goenka, the founder of the centre. He was very cordial and remembered our meeting when I was in India. I requested him to consider Kevin for the next course, starting in a week's time. He was gracious enough to accede to my request. I helped him book his travel from Mumbai airport to Igatpuri and connected him to some of my contacts in Mumbai.

Kevin was ready for his transformation.

## 13

'We have begun our descent into Mumbai. Hope you had a pleasant flight. Thank you for flying Singapore Airlines,' the pilot's voice woke me up.

The lovely smile of the air hostess greeted me as I opened my eyes. It took me a while to realise that Myanmar and Kevin were a distant but pleasant memory.

I allowed myself to think them for one last time. 'Om Namah Shivay,' I said to myself and smiled.

After the Vipassana course, Kevin was indeed a transformed man. He kept coming to me once a month. When he would come, he would lie on the therapy chair and go to sleep. In a short while, he would also be snoring. After thirty minutes, he would wake up and speak his mind. There was so much clarity in his thoughts now. I would ask him why was paying me for these sessions when all he did was come and sleep.

He would say, 'Dr Pandit, I feel a sense of calm here. This is the couch which connected me back with my life, and if possible, I want to take it with me.'

We would have a hearty laugh.

He gracefully separated from his girlfriend, Vivian. He stopped his trips to Bangkok, and for many months, he was actually single. His renewed focus on the business helped, and it started growing which also increased his confidence.

As the plane touched down at Mumbai airport, I had smile on my face.

# CHAPTER 4

# SWAN SOARING IN THE SKY

## 1

My name is Fei Hong. When I was six years old, I lived in a small village called Qixin, which is one of the most backward areas of Guizhao province, in rural China.

I lived there with my father, Wang Wei, and mother, Yu Yan. They were a typical hardworking couple who struggled through the day to make ends meet.

To me, they are the world. My father was the kindest person you will ever meet, and my mother the most beautiful. My mother's smile was as beautiful as her name suggests. She was my hero.

My mother would wake up at 5 a.m. every day and start her journey, on foot, with other women of our village to the nearest source of water, which was about 7 miles away. This was the early 1980s, and while the world beyond our village was in the throes of economic development, electricity was still unheard of in Qixin. In the darkness, the women would find their way on a dirt road strewn with pebbles. My mother would carry two buckets fastened to either end of yoke-like shoulder poles, which would be filled with water on the way back. Upon returning from this arduous journey, she would cook food and then go to the paddy fields and join my father, who would have already spent a few hours there.

That day was just like any other typical day in our lives. Or that's what we thought.

I woke up early to find my mother about to leave the tiny mud dwelling, which was our house. I did not want her to go and so started crying. She gave her sweet smile and took me in her arms.

'My *baobei*, what's the matter?' she said lovingly.

'Mùnǎiyī,' I muttered in between my tears, 'please don't go today.'

'I have to go,' she said while running her fingers gently through my hair, 'else Mùnǎiyī will not be able to cook yummy rice cakes for her *baobei*.'

She kissed me gently. I just wanted to be in her arms. It felt so warm.

Neither of us however, had a choice.

She took the pole with the two buckets, looked at me once again, and left. Her lovely smile seemed so much brighter in the flicker of the oil lamp in the corner.

I felt her warmth beside me as I gently drifted back to sleep.

'Fei Hong,' the sound of my name being called out woke me up. I opened my eyes and looked around. Sunlight was streaming in from the small hole in the wall. The lady from our next house was calling my name.

'Fei Hong,' she said hurriedly, 'please come with me.'

'Where is Mùnǎiyī,' I asked.

She did not answer but held my hand and almost dragged me out of the house. We kept walking on the muddy path. My feet were hurting, and I was scared.

'I want my Mùnǎiyī,' I kept pleading in between my tears.

We finally reached a small building, which I recognised as the place where my mother had brought me a few days ago when I was sick. There were people gathered outside and many of them came forward and held my hand or patted my head. My six-year-old brain could not fathom what was happening.

Inside that building, the lady took me to one of the rooms, and there I finally saw my father.

'Fùqīn,' I screamed with joy and ran to him.

'My *baobei*,' he said and took me in his arms.

I realised that he was crying as he hugged me tightly.

With my tiny fingers, I tried to wipe his tears, but they just wouldn't stop.

He slowly gathered himself and spoke to me.

'My *baobei*,' he said softly, 'your Mùnǎiyī is not well. Tell her she will be all right.'

He guided me to the bed, and there I saw my mother.

'Mùnǎiyī,' I screamed with joy and jumped on the bed with her.

She was sitting in a hunched position with her face between her knees. Hearing my voice, she looked up.

Her hair was messy, and her eyes were swollen. Her clothes were torn, and there was blood on her arms. The smile was nowhere to be seen.

I cuddled myself into her arms, but her hands were limp. I took her hands and guided them to my cheeks which she would pull fondly, but her fingers remained lifeless.

She did not speak to me, but I remained there until my father took me out of the room. We sat outside as people rushed in and out of the room.

I did not know what was happening, but I had a feeling that something was wrong … terribly wrong.

I saw my mother again only in the evening. Some ladies brought her home. They kept telling her, 'Everything will be OK,' but my mother was silent. She did not speak a word. In fact, I had not heard her voice since the time she left the house in the morning.

I went to my father and whispered, 'What happened to Mùnǎiyī?'

'Some evil people have hurt her,' he said softly. 'She is in pain. We have to take care of her.'

'I will take care of her,' I announced.

I had not eaten anything that day, and I was hungry. Something had happened to my dear Mùnǎiyī and I had to take care of her. I did not tell her that I was hungry; nor did I pester her to tell me a story. All I wanted was to see her smile.

I lay in the corner and kept looking at her. Her eyes were just staring at the plain wall in front of her. My father was sitting next to her with his head between his knees. I had never seen them so sad.

The night, I had a dream. My mother was cuddling me. She was pulling my chubby cheeks and singing a song for me. She was telling stories of the little princess who lives in this lovely castle. I was so happy to finally see her smile.

I was jolted out of my sleep again by someone calling my name.

It was the same lady who had woken me up the previous night. She held my hand and took me out. This time it was only a short walk. In the darkness, I could see the old well near our house. I was told that this well was deep and the water poisonous. My older friends would tell me that it was haunted. My mother would warn me not to go near it. I felt scared and held on to the lady's hand tightly.

And then I saw her ...

She was lying on the ground ... motionless. People were standing around her. I ran to her. She was covered in a pool of blood. Her face was unrecognisable, her wet clothes in tatters and her hands cold ... really cold.

'Mùnǎiyī,' I called, 'please wake up.'

There was no response. I started crying and looked around for my father. There he was, a few feet away, crying hysterically.

*What is happening?* I wondered. Until yesterday, everyone was so happy. But now everyone seemed to be so sad. My father was crying, all the time and my dear Mùnǎiyī had not spoken to me for so long.

'Fei Hong,' I heard someone call my name. It was the grand old lady of the village. She held me close to her and said, 'You dear Mùnǎiyī has gone to the heavens up there and has become an angel.'

I could not understand.

'I want my Mùnǎiyī,' I cried.

'Fei Hong, you Mùnǎiyī has left us. However, when you think of her, you will feel her near you. She will love you just as she was doing before.'

'I want my Mùnǎiyī,' I wailed even louder.

But that was never going to happen. I would never see the lovely smile again. The big bad world had taken away the most precious thing I had.

**2**

'Life isn't about finding yourself. Life is about creating yourself.'

This famous quote by George Bernard Shaw has been a huge influence in my life. Very often, we flow with the tide, letting life take us to the unknown. Rather than just living every moment, I believe in making things happen and bringing life to every moment. I ensure that I keep myself involved in pursuits which occupy my body and mind in equal measure. Yoga and meditation early in the morning rejuvenates me and fills me with the energy to go through the day. In the evenings, I take a walk or go for a jog. On some days, it is swimming, and on others, it may be a game of tennis.

I am at the One°15 Marina club today and have planned a game of tennis with a very special person. I have always maintained my distance with every client of mine. The relationship remains strictly formal during our engagement and beyond. Some of my clients do keep in touch with me on the internet but the conversations remain within the boundaries I have drawn for myself. The person I am meeting today is possibly the only exception. She was in the troughs of her career, relationship, health, and life in general when she met me for the first time. By helping her find the true purpose in life and encouraging her at every step, I saw her experience a transformation that very few others have achieved. Over the period, we developed a bond which transformed our formal relationship into one of friendship. She is based in Singapore, and so we do manage to catch up once every few months.

At the club, I changed into my tennis gear and headed to the courts. The club has two outdoor hardcourt tennis courts with acrylic surface sand. There was a game in progress on both the courts. I sat down on one of the chairs and gently placed my rather heavy kit by my side. The doubles game was being played at a frenetic pace, and the four men were in high spirits as they pumped their fists and cheered every winner.

'Hello, Dr Preeti,' a sweet voice called from behind me.

I turned around to see her with a big grin on her face and with her hands held wide.

'Hello, Vivian.' I stood up and gave her a warm hug.

She was wearing a lovely white skirt and sleeveless top. She sported a Nike headband to keep her short hair in place.

'So good to see you,' I said, and she reciprocated with a 'same here'.

I directed her to the chair next to the one I was sitting on.

'How have you been?' I asked as she settled down and opened her kit bag.

'Dr Preeti, I have been well,' she said with the smile still intact. 'In fact things could not be better.'

I noticed more than a tinge of excitement in her voice.

'Good to hear that,' I responded and enquired, 'Anything interesting to share?'

'I do,' she replied and then paused. 'I will leave it for the postgame drink.'

The sudden surge in the noise level from the court diverted my attention. One of the pairs had won, and the winners were celebrating boisterously. After the shaking of hands across the net, the four men came off the court laughing and mimicking some of their shots. It was good to see this kind of sportsmanship and reminded me of a phrase by a sporting icon: 'I don't have enemies. Only opponents.'

'Let's play?' I enquired and stood up.

'Just a minute,' Vivian said as she finished her routine of tightening the strings of her racquet, having a few sips of water, removing a towel, and keeping it ready for use during the game. I smiled, as I had done precisely the same things a few minutes ago.

We had a wonderful game which lasted for about an hour. The sweat on my brow and the wet towels suggested that we had a good workout.

After a quick shower, we settled down at the coffee shop for a cup of iced tea.

'So, Vivian,' I said, 'I am waiting to hear the interesting news.'

'I have been promoted to the role of a manager,' she blurted out with a scream.

Vivian was working in a multinational bank in the HR function. After the low in her life and career over the last five years, she had been making sincere efforts to get back into the mainstream and resurrect her career. This was a real sign of an upswing.

'That's wonderful,' I responded and extended my hand to congratulate her.

She held my hand with both hands and paused as she looked into my eyes.

'I cannot thank you enough, Dr Preeti,' she said softly.

I responded with a smile of reassurance.

'Career has always been important for me, but I got entangled in a web, probably of my own creation,' she continued. 'And it was you who helped me untangle myself. I must confess that I did put a lot of efforts during the year. This promotion is a just reward.'

She seemed so happy and full of life.

Who would believe that about three years ago, this was the same lady who had been in police custody for violent behaviour in public?

# 3

*Three years earlier …*

'Hello, Dr Pandit,' the voice on the phone said. 'This is Officer James Carter from Nanyang Neighbourhood Police Centre.'

The name and the voice seemed familiar.

'I am Dr Pandit,' I responded hesitantly.

'We have met before,' the officer said, 'for the case of Miss Vivian Chang.'

*Oh … that's why the voice sounded familiar*, I thought. He did not have to remind me about that incident.

'Yes,' I responded.

'Well … we need your presence at the centre again,' he remarked.

'What's the matter?' I asked, fearing the worst.

'We have Miss Vivian Chang in our custody again,' he replied, 'and we need you to testify.'

'Oh!' was all I could muster.

'If you are ready, I could send a patrol car to bring you here,' he offered.

I looked at the clock on the wall in front of me. It was nearing 7 p.m. Pankaj was away in Malaysia, and I did not have anything planned for the evening.

'Yes, please,' I replied.

At the police station, the handsome officer shook my hand and thanked me for coming at such short notice.

'Miss Vivian Chang was at the Orchard Central Mall, where she had an altercation with an attendant at one of the stores,' he narrated. 'Apparently, she was hysterical and could have caused some serious harm if the other attendants had not intervened and restrained her. The store manager lodged a complaint, and we had to bring her to the station.'

I shook my head in despair.

'I checked our records and found an earlier complaint registered against her,' the officer continued. 'The records also state that she was released based on your statement of her mental condition.'

'Yes, Officer,' I said without getting into the details.

He continued, 'We can release her on one condition …'

He paused. I waited in anticipation.

'You have to take her for therapy,' the officer said after some thought.

I usually accept a case only after I have evaluated the readiness of the client. I firmly believe that any therapy will work only when the subject is ready and believes in the process. I did not seem to have the luxury of that evaluation here if I had to help the lady.

'I will do that,' I agreed without too much of a thought, as the sensitive part of me took over.

The officer summoned Vivian from the other room.

'Please sit down, miss,' he beckoned her to the chair in front of him.

Vivian was in tears. I could see her feet trembling as she took the support of the table while sitting down.

'Miss Vivian Chang,' the officer said, 'the manager of the store has lodged a complaint against you. This is the second time that you have caused a disturbance in public. Do you agree?'

'Yes, Officer,' Vivian said, barely managing to control her tears.

The officer continued, 'I would like to put it on record that if we receive another complaint of similar nature, we will need to charge you and produce you in court.'

'Yes, Officer,' she responded.

The officer continued, 'Since the two complaints pointed to a possible mental condition, I will also put it on record that you have been advised therapy. Do you agree to undergo therapy?'

'Yes, Officer,' she repeated.

The officer pointed in my direction and said to Vivian, 'You know Dr Pandit?'

She raised her head a little to look at me and nodded. 'Yes, I do.'

'Do you agree to undergo therapy with her?' he asked with authority.

'Yes, Officer,' she replied more clearly as she slowly got hold of herself.

Officer James Carter then addressed me.

'Dr Pandit, would you be ready to sign an undertaking about her mental health?' he asked.

I looked at the dishevelled figure of Vivian and nodded.

'We will also request you to inform the police station if Miss Vivian Chang does not start her therapy in a week's time,' he added.

'OK, Officer!' I agreed.

The officer completed the formalities and thanked me for coming to the station. I gave my business card to Vivian and asked her to call me the next day.

# 4

Vivian called the next day and fixed an appointment for the day after.

She was punctual. She was wearing a black skirt and a pink floral top. Her long hair was let loose. Her fair skin complemented the dark lipstick she was wearing. Her shoulders were broad, like those of a sportsperson. She had a pleasant personality completely, unlike what I had seen at the police centre.

'Hello, Dr Pandit.' She bowed in a typical Chinese gesture. 'Thank you for helping me at the police centre.'

I smiled at her and said, 'Vivian. I am a therapist. I can see the real Vivian hidden inside the person I saw at the police centre and also the person sitting in front of me.' I leaned forward and looked in her eyes. 'Vivian, if you want to, we can set that person free. Are you ready?'

I could see tears welling in her eyes. She folded her hands. Her words came out in gasps. 'My life is a mess, Dr Pandit. I don't know what's happened to me. I need your help.'

'I am here to guide you,' I assured her, 'but you have to first believe in the process and then do whatever is required. Change is simple, but it is not easy. It may be very difficult to break the old habits which are controlling your life. But once you do that, your life will be what you always wanted it to be. Are you ready to take up this challenge?'

There was a twinkle in her eye, which was a sign to me that she wanted to go through this process of transformation. I had my answer and what she said now did not matter.

'I am willing to do whatever is needed to set myself free.'

'Good,' I acknowledged her resolve. 'Let's begin.'

I looked at her. With the dark circles around her eyes, she looked much older than her thirty-four years.

'Vivian, please can you move to that chair,' I said, pointing to the therapy chair in one corner of the room.

Once settled, I started the session.

'Vivian, when you are comfortable please close your eyes. Let your breathing come to normal,' I said softly.

I gave her some time.

'I invite you to reflect on your life. Look at your life as if you are watching a movie. Bring the memories of your life into the movie and let me know what you see,' I said.

She remained silent, but I could sense that she was going deep within herself. And then the floodgates opened.

'I am struck in this web, and as I keep trying harder, I seem to be getting entangled even more. My boyfriend is in a state of panic, as he cannot do anything about the situation that I am facing. He sees that I am pushing him to do the things that he does not want to do, yet he knows that it will make me upset if he doesn't do it, and I will push until he gives in. I am stubborn and adamant. Yet he cannot leave me because he knows I will be upset so he feels struck in this relationship. He is worried for me because he loves me. His perception of love towards me is that of obligation and concern.'

She paused. I could see from her expressions that she was getting uncomfortable.

'Probably, the romantic love that we had has diminished. It appears he is helpless and difficult because it involves a lot of sacrifice of his own priorities and beliefs. He feels he is being pushed too much. And yet, he has no way out. He wants to be around for me to be well, but I keep making things very difficult for him. He feels that he has to deal with so many problems in life apart from me as well. His perception of love is that he wants me to be well, and yet he wants to do his own things. He perceives love between us now to be very miserable because it is making things difficult for him and causing him a lot of stress. He knows that either he sacrifices his life, or he discontinues this relationship and gives me up. And I am the cause of his stress.'

She started trembling. Her head started shaking, and she seemed in a lot of visible discomfort.

'I am the reason for the mess that we are in,' she screamed and sat up on the chair.

She started weeping loudly and started pulling her hair in disgust.

'Vivian,' I called out authoritatively. 'Vivian, come back to the present.'

It took a while for her to calm down. She raised her head slowly from her cupped hands. I extended the tissue box, which she gladly accepted. A few wet tissues later, she seemed in control, at least for the moment.

'Vivian, do you practise meditation?' I asked.

'No,' she muttered, 'but my boyfriend does a lot of it.'

'I will teach you a few simple breathing techniques, which I want you to do every morning. Start with fifteen minutes, and slowly increase it to thirty minutes,' I explained.

I gave her a demonstration and asked her to repeat the same until I was convinced that she had understood.

I bid her goodbye and fixed a date and time for the next session in the following week.

Vivian seemed to be blaming herself for the relationship with her boyfriend going sour. She also seemed afraid of losing him. There were a lot of things bottled up inside her which needed a release.

## 5

She walked in with a smile, a complete contrast to how she had left my clinic the other day. Her formal pants and jacket made her look elegant. She greeted me and took her position on the therapy chair.

'How are the breathing exercises helping?' I asked.

She smiled sheepishly. 'I did it for a couple of days but could not continue.'

'Did someone stop you from doing it?' I asked without hiding my annoyance.

'Er ... no, Dr Pandit,' she said sullenly.

'You were blaming yourself for your situation last week,' I said impassively, 'and I feel you were right. I had asked you to commit fifteen minutes a day, but you could not even manage that. I think you are comfortable with your life, even if what you say may seem otherwise.'

A thought, word, or action when repeated multiple times with similar outcomes becomes ingrained in our mind, and it becomes difficult to dissociate them from the outcomes. An event which did not go well for us may trigger a thought: *I am not good*. When a few such events happen in quick succession, this thought, *I am not good enough*, becomes ingrained in our heads. This simple thought, if not controlled, in time, can play havoc in our lives, as we quickly start doubting our own abilities in everything we do. Breaking this pattern is not easy since it requires a more powerful positive thought to replace this belief, and for that positive thought to become powerful requires many conscious repetitions. We get so used to the negative patterns that breaking them requires a lot of disciplined effort.

It was this discipline that I wanted to instil in Vivian, since we had a long way to go and I wanted her to get into good habits quickly.

My tirade made the right impact.

Vivian appeared crestfallen, which was unfortunate but necessary.

'I am sorry, Dr Pandit,' she apologised, 'I will not give you any reason to be disappointed with me again.' She appeared sincere.

I remained silent and allowed her to feel repentant for a little while longer.

'Where do you work Vivian?' I enquired.

She was working as an office assistant at a local company in District 15. The company was in the IT products and services business. She had joined a month ago. Apparently, this was her third job in the last six months.

'Can we move to the chair?' I asked, pointing to the therapy chair.

Once she was one with herself, I asked her, 'Vivian, I want you to visualise the life of your dreams. Look into the future and see yourself living that life. Your life is all that you wanted it to be.'

I wanted her to see something that she may not have seen before. I watched as her body started responding.

'What do you see, Vivian?' I asked softly.

'The sky is clouded. There is a storm coming. Everything is so dark. People are rushing to their homes. It's very windy. Things are flying all over the place. I am trying to hold on. There is no one to help me. I am all alone. People are dying. There is blood all over.' The words were coming out wistfully, and I had to intervene.

'Vivian, the storm will clear one day,' I said firmly, wanting to reassure her, 'Things will fall into place. You will do well in your career. You will have people with you. I want you to look beyond the storm. I want you to enter this world where things are happening exactly the way you would have wanted.'

We are more likely to succeed in a task when we set a goal. The goal creates an anticipation, it creates a belief, it creates hope. By urging her to visualise her dream, I was helping her set a goal for herself. The therapy would help her reach that goal. I wanted to create the anticipation of a new life, a life that she would have forgotten about while grappling with her present situation.

It took me a while, but it happened. There was a hint of a smile on her lips.

'I am so happy ... I am in this big office, and everyone is applauding me for something ... Yes, I see my name on the door of the cabin ... There is a big table, and behind me is a glass wall from where I can see the Singapore skyline,' she said slowly.

She was now beginning to enjoy the moments being played out in her mind's eye.

'That's wonderful,' I said encouragingly. 'You had a lovely day at work. Where are you going after work?' I asked, wanting to understand where her thoughts were leading her.

She shook her head, probably sifting through the many thoughts in her head.

'I have this beautiful house. It's a large apartment ... There is a lovely sofa unit in the living room ... The kitchen is spacious, with all the cutlery properly arranged in white cabinets ... There is a library with lots of books and an armchair next to a lovely reading lamp ...' She paused at this point, probably seeing herself in that armchair with a book in hand.

'The bedroom is full of soft toys, and the walls have paintings of babies on them.' She was unhurried as she shared the details.

I was letting her live a few moments, which were probably in stark contrast to her present life, and she was enjoying them.

'Who is there with you in the house?' I asked slowly, not wanting to disturb her thoughts but wanting to get some hint into her relationships.

She remained silent. She was probably searching for someone.

After a brief moment, a smile returned to her lips. This time it was more pronounced.

'My little baby. She is so cute … She has curly hair … She is looking so innocent as she sleeps … I feel like cuddling her in my arms and …'

She stopped. Her expressions changed suddenly as if she had just woken up from a dream.

She opened her eyes and looked around, trying to figure out where she was. And then the tears started flowing. She held her face in her hands and sobbed uncontrollably. She had been jolted back to reality.

I had achieved my objective. I had given her the hope of a better life. I had anchored her to a goal.

I thought things would start getting better now.

I was badly mistaken.

# 6

I was in the clinic, reading one of my case files, when Sandra peeped in.

'Dr Pandit, there is a call for you from the company Excel Limited,' she said. 'Shall I connect?'

That did not ring a bell. I don't like to be disturbed when I am preparing for a session.

'Can you please take a message?' I suggested. 'I am in the middle of something.'

'I already tried doing that,' she replied, 'but the gentleman insisted that its important.'

I had no choice.

'Am I speaking with Dr Pandit?' the voice at the other end enquired.

'Yes, I am Dr Pandit,' I replied searchingly. 'Who is this?'

'My name is Peter May,' the person said. 'I am the HR manager at Excel Limited. I need to speak to you about Miss Vivian Chang.'

*Oh no. Not again* was the thought that crossed my mind as soon as I heard the name.

'Go ahead,' I said.

'Vivian is our employee, and she has been causing a lot of trouble in the office,' he said. 'We issued a termination letter to her today when she told us that she is not well and is undergoing therapy with you. I want to confirm if that's true.'

In all my years of practice, I have never been required to keep testifying for any of my clients like I was doing now.

'Mr May,' I said slowly, 'I am a psychotherapist, and Miss Vivian Chang is indeed my client.'

'Dr Pandit,' he said in a tone which suggested he was not in the best of moods, 'it is my duty to inform you that Miss Chang has been a troublemaker at work. She picks up a fight with her colleagues for petty reasons and has been regularly found abusing some of them.'

'I am sorry, Mr May,' I said. 'I am sorry for her behaviour. She is indeed going through a very difficult time in her life. I am helping her get things sorted.'

'Dr Pandit,' he said in a more apologetic tone this time, 'considering her medical condition, I will take back the termination letter but with a warning. I hope that you will be able to help her get better.'

'Thank you for your consideration, Mr May,' I said, feeling relieved. 'I do hope that she gets better soon.'

'Thank you, Dr Pandit,' he said and ended the call.

I shook my head as I sat back on my chair. Vivian had been let off with a warning by the police twice and now by her employer. Vivian needed help, and she needed it immediately.

I decided that I would have two sessions with her every week instead of the standard one session that I have with my clients. It was also clear that I would need to take some immediate measures to calm her down. Much against my belief, I consulted a psychiatrist and requested that he prescribe some mild antianxiety drugs. Desperate situations require desperate measures, and this was one of them.

# 7

Over the next few sessions, I tried different therapies on Vivian.

Her whole life was revolving around her boyfriend, Kevin, who also happened to be my client. He was having issues with his life for which he was undergoing therapy. It was necessary to know Vivian's side of the story.

'How did you meet your boyfriend?' I asked her when we started one of our sessions.

'One morning, as I was walking down the stairway of my apartment block, he was a few feet ahead of me. All of a sudden, he collapsed. I rushed to help him. He seemed to have lost consciousness. I called the emergency services, and they helped him to a hospital. When he was back in his apartment, I went to visit him a few times.'

'When did you develop some feelings for him?' I enquired.

She continued, 'He seemed a nice person. I realised that he was alone, and I offered to help. I would prepare soup for him. When I visited him, we used to have long conversations. He would share stories of his life. He described in detail about his love for his ex-wife, Rachel. He would talk so much about her. I would always wonder how someone can love another person so much. He talked about how difficult his life was after she left him. He would talk about the Hindu god Shiva and his influence. I would sit and listen to him, enamoured by his love for another person. I would look forward to spending more time in his apartment. I did not know how and when it happened, but I developed an infatuation for him—his handsome personality and his warmth.'

She paused.

I remained silent waiting for her to gather her thoughts.

'What did you do about it?' I prodded.

She recollected, 'I was not sure what I should be doing. This was the first time I had felt something like this. All I wanted was to be with him. It was his birthday. I baked a cake for him. I wanted the day to be special for him. He was looking so handsome in his jacket. After he cut the cake, he leaned forward and kissed me. I did not resist. He was so gentle. I had never been kissed so softly. All I wanted was to be with him.'

'Everything seemed good,' I said. 'What happened?'

'I feel that I am not worthy of him,' she replied dolefully.

'And what made you think that?' I probed.

'He has so many friends and has such an exciting life, while mine is boring and I'm still engaged in having to make ends meet and having work as my main focus. His life goals are now travelling, meeting people, and just enjoying life. I want him to be with me all the time. I want to hold him and hear him talk, but he is so busy in his work.'

'Doesn't he spend time with you now?' I enquired.

She cringed as she spoke.

'I so look forward to his coming home from his business travels. I cook food for him, and I dream of all the things I want to talk to him about. All I want him to do is sit with me for some time and talk to me. Tell me about his trip. But he just eats his food and goes to bed. I wish he would at least ask me if I have eaten.'

I could see the little teardrops in her eyes.

She continued, 'Maybe he is tired and I am expecting too much from him. I try not to talk about heavy subjects with him all the time. I try to make every moment with him, an enjoyable and relaxing one—by giving him enough space and time to do the things that he wants and not to bother him by continuously communicating with him.'

This was a different perspective to the same situation. For Kevin, this need of Vivian seemed like overpossessiveness and was driving him away from her. The more she tried, the more he was moving away.

'Maybe he is really busy at work and it is making him tired,' I said, recollecting my conversations with Kevin. 'This happens in every relationship. We have to find the right time and space for a conversation.'

'Hmmm,' she mused, 'but I don't know if I am good enough for him.'

'What makes you think that?' I asked again.

She covered her face with her hands.

'And what Vivian?' I prodded her.

She fell silent and continued to stare at the floor.

This was a very crucial information for Kevin's case and gave me a lead to follow.

'Vivian, I want you to bring out every feeling, every emotion that you have in this relationship,' I assured her. 'Saying what you feel doesn't make you bad. In fact, it will only help you see your life differently.'

I was giving her the space she felt she never had. And she made the most of it.

'He gets physically touchy with other girls. He rubs their backs and touches their waist. He flirts back with whoever flirts with him. He does not show any self-restraint.'

Her insecurities were slowly finding an expression.

'He has dubious relations with married women. Not sexual or anything, just very unusually close. They may be close friends, but he tells me stories that these women used to like him or used to be lovers, but they still keep in touch and he gets a lot of special attention from them ... He even confessed he would visit prostitutes ... He is very secretive. When he comes back from his travels, he messages the friends whom he has met, mostly girls, younger ones ... Thanks for your company, enjoyed it a lot. See you next time ... He visits different friends each time he travels, but he tells me only of certain friends, mostly male, that he visits. He does not tell me of others. But I find out later that he is meeting many of his female friends during his overseas trips.'

The little tears now turned into a flood and the sobs turned into loud wails. She was hysterical, probably feeling guilty for harbouring these feelings.

It took a while for her to regain control, but I was sure that she must be feeling so much lighter than when she walked in that day.

Vivian had fallen head over heels in love with Kevin. When Kevin reciprocated, it was as if all her dreams had come true. She always had a sense of insecurity about the relationship because, in her mind, she was so ordinary in comparison to Kevin's almost flamboyant personality. She was ready to ignore all the indiscretions of Kevin as long as he was with her. But some corner of her mind was asking for more from him. The insecurity made her increasingly possessive, but to her conscious self, she just wanted to spend more time with him. All she wanted was for Kevin to reciprocate and show the desire to be with her, which never happened. She kept supressing this want, but beyond a point, Kevin's rejections of her many advances started manifesting in the anxiety attacks and hysterical behaviour. That probably explained the incidents for which I was called to the police station.

I had many clients who were going through a tough time in their life due to their possessiveness but none who would get into a state of hysteria that Vivian exhibited.

There must be a trigger; in most cases, it is events from the past. I had to delve into her past. More precisely, I wanted her to identify the incidents from her past which had probably led to her present behaviour.

## 8

When we met again, I initiated the conversation.

'Vivian,' I said softly, 'our present behaviour is influenced a lot by our environment when we were kids. In that impressionable age, certain beliefs get ingrained in us which either surfaces sometime later in life or remain in some deep, dark corner of the mind and don't allow our best self to come forward.'

Vivian was listening attentively.

'I want to do a hypnotherapy session with you to help you get into these deep dark corners of your mind and crush these thoughts and beliefs which are a stumbling block in your life,' I explained.

She seemed willing to do whatever was necessary to gift herself a brighter future.

In about twenty minutes, she was in her past.

'Where are you, Vivian?' I asked.

'I am in Singapore, living in a home for children,' she muttered slowly.

'Who brought you here?' I enquired.

'An old man. He is telling me that these people will take care of me,' she replied haltingly.

'How old are you?' I asked.

'I think … 10 years.'

'I want you to go further back in time and tell me, who is this old man?' I quizzed 'Please ask him.'

'He is a kind man. He is taking me, in a plane. He is giving me nice food,' she jogged her memory.

'Where is he taking you? Please ask him.'

'To Singapore,' she replied.

'Where are you now?' I asked.

'In Shanghai.'

'Tell me more about what you are doing in Shanghai,' I asked, trying to help her trace a path through her past.

She fell silent.

I waited for a few minutes and prodded her 'Vivian, you are in Shanghai. What are you seeing?'

All of a sudden, her body started writhing in visible discomfort.

I held her hand and went close to her ear. 'Vivian, it's OK,' I assured her. 'I am with you. Don't be afraid. Tell me what you see.'

'He is dead,' she screamed.

'Who?' I asked softly.

She was still in the past and was seeing something which was causing this hysterical response. 'My father,' she bellowed.

'How did he die?' I continued.

'Accident … The old man says there was an accident in the factory,' she said poignantly.

As I helped her revisit her past, she narrated that she was living with her father in Shanghai. After the tragic accident, the old man brought her from Shanghai to Singapore and enrolled her into a children's home here.

'The world is a cruel place. It is taking away all the people I love' were her final words before she broke down uncontrollably. I had to bring her back to the present.

Vivian seemed to have had a difficult childhood. She had seen her father die in an accident, and an old man had brought her to Singapore and put her in a children's home.

Who was the old man? What about her mother? What did her last statement mean?

I could not find the answers to these questions for a few weeks since Vivian's relationship with Kevin was getting worse and our sessions were focussed on reducing her growing anxiety.

And then, the sessions with Kevin took a different turn.

It was now clear that Vivian's possessiveness was driving Kevin away from her. Kevin was never in love with Vivian in the first place. It was his obsession with his ex-wife Rachel that made him see her image in Vivian. But Vivian's efforts to be with him all the time were driving him away. As they drifted apart, he started to find solace in other women who resembled Rachel in some aspect. Unlike what Vivian assumed, he had never committed himself to her.

Although it was never my objective, I would now have to make Vivian realise the fact that there had been no relationship at all. She was clinging onto a person for whom she did not actually exist.

# 9

It had been more than a month since the hypnotherapy session. I decided that It was now time to look ahead and get her life back in order. I would come back to seek answers to some of my questions from her past sometime later. A little detail had caught my attention from one of the earlier sessions. I planned to do something with it.

'Vivian, what book are you reading now?' I asked when she came for her next session.

She seemed to be taken aback by the question.

'Book?' she asked and responded, 'Nothing in particular.'

'Why is that? You love books, don't you?' I queried.

Her face lit up.

'Yes, Dr Pandit,' she said. 'I used to be a voracious reader in my younger days. In fact, books were my best companion, but … now I don't get the time.'

'What keeps you busy, Vivian?' I asked with a faint smile.

She was at a loss to answer that question.

'I don't know …' she thought aloud.

'That's OK. Don't think too much about it,' I assured her. 'Why don't we transport you to your younger years and get you into the reading habit again?'

She started beaming from ear to ear. It was as if a child had been promised her favourite toy. This was the happiest I had seen Vivian since the last few weeks that I had been working with her. I felt assured that I was moving in the right direction.

'What time do you leave from work?' I asked.

'Around 5 p.m.,' she said.

'What do you do once you are back at home?'

'I cook dinner, watch some television, and …' She tried figuring out something more. 'Sometimes I go shopping for groceries.'

I interrupted her and asked, 'You mentioned earlier that your office is in District 15, right? That is not too far away from East Coast Park.'

She nodded.

'OK, this is what I want you to do,' I told her. 'Every evening after you leave the office, get to the East Coast Park. Find a silent part of the beach, sit on the sand, and read a book for one hour. Is that possible?' I asked.

'Yes,' she blurted without a second thought.

'When can you start?' I enquired.

'Today,' she said, and her voice was full of excitement.

'That's wonderful.' I smiled in acknowledgement. 'Here, this is my gift to you,' I said and handed the book that I had bought for her.

She almost jumped up from her chair.

'*The Alchemist*,' she read the title. 'I have heard so much about this book.' She looked at me and said, 'Thank you so much, Dr Pandit.'

'Most welcome, Vivian,' I said, acknowledging her show of gratitude, and added, 'When you come here for your next session, we will have a discussion on the book. Is that OK?'

'Most definitely,' she said. 'I would be very happy to do that.'

From that day, the sessions were primarily focussed on the books she was reading and the messages that she was able to get from them. I suggested books like the autobiography of Helen Keller (*The Story of My Life*) and the autobiography of Oprah Winfrey, among others. The idea was to show her the challenges that other people have faced and not only overcome but used as a springboard to attain great heights.

Book psychotherapy is a technique used to inspire positivity in the mindsets of affected people and help them live better lives. Those who experience depression or anxiety can be low on energy and enthusiasm for a long time. When the body is relaxed through meditation, positive thoughts and actions can result and lead to positive change. Meditative practice combined with creative experience, such as book psychotherapy, can enable patients to process their emotions and begin to enjoy life. Book psychotherapy under proper guidance from a psychotherapist provides the opportunity to speed up healing, transformation, and personal growth.

Vivian was indeed a voracious reader. She would read for an hour initially, but that increased to almost two hours on many days. She would finish a book in less than a week, so we were discussing a new book in almost every session. It was wonderful to note that after she went back to her reading habit, there were hardly any sessions where she came to me with her problems. On the contrary, there would be at least one learning that she would take away from every session. I taught her some breathing and meditation techniques which she could practise at home.

In a few weeks, there was a visible improvement in Vivian. Importantly, there were no further distress calls for me, and even more importantly, she continued in the same job. In consultation with the psychiatrist, I asked her to stop the medicines she was having.

However, her personal life was getting into even stormier waters.

## 10

'I want to end this relationship,' Kevin stated the now obvious to Vivian after another bitter argument.

Their relationship had deteriorated over the past few months, although the frequency and the intensity of the arguments had significantly reduced thanks to the therapy sessions that they were undergoing. The therapy was not focussed on their relationship but was expected to help them see their situation from multiple perspectives and to handle it maturely.

Actually, the seeds of separation were sown long before the therapies commenced. In fact, from Kevin's point of view, their relationship only existed in the fantasy world that he was living in, and it ceased to exist when he started coming back to reality.

Vivian was heartbroken. Despite all that she was going through, she had given everything to this relationship. She had never loved someone so deeply.

'Kevin, I truly love you,' she managed to say through the tears. 'We can still make this work.'

'I want to believe that I loved you as well,' Kevin confessed, 'but I now realise that it was not the case. I have gotten over Rachel now, and I have wanted to experience this newfound freedom for some time.'

Vivian wouldn't let go.

'Everything there was between us cannot just be a fantasy.' She was wailing now. 'I promise to give you the freedom that you want. I realise that I may not have given you the space you wanted. Believe me, I am changing. The therapy is working.'

She was literally clinging onto Kevin and almost pleading now.

Kevin did not resist; nor did he try to calm her down.

She cried until her throat was dry and her voice was coarse. With very little energy left, she slid down his body and slumped at his feet. She remained on the floor as Kevin gathered some of his stuff and left the apartment.

They would never meet each other.

She broke down again as she narrated the incident during our session.

She appeared heartbroken and sad, which was a natural response to the situation she was in (unlike the possible hysterical behaviour she would otherwise have exhibited).

I told her a quote by the famous poet Khalil Gibran: 'If you love somebody, let them go, for if they return, they were always yours. And if they don't, they never were.'

'It was never meant to be,' I advised Vivian when she had calmed down. 'Let out your emotions. Cry as much as you want. But when the tears stop, you need to take stock of the situation. You have been progressing towards your goal very well. Let this incident not come in the way of a better life for yourself.'

These words had a calming effect on her. She used the last of the tissues, sniffed, and sat upright on the chair.

'I agree, Dr Pandit,' she stated. 'Please tell me what I should be doing.'

'I want you to tell the universe about the life you want to lead,' I told her. 'The law of attraction states that the universe is abundant in its riches. However, you need to ask for what you desire. You need to ask not just with words, but you should also mean it through every nerve of your body. That's when you will be vibrating at a frequency where you will be open to receiving.'

I gave her a writing pad and a pencil.

'Vivian,' I said softly, 'I invite you to ask the universe whatever you desire. Bring those desires to the fore and write them down.'

I had done a future-pacing exercise with her earlier, but her perspective of life was very different then. With all the reading she had been doing, her outlook was bound to be more positive.

She put her mind to the task and started writing. She was asking the universe for a better life, the life of her dreams.

It was a good thirty-five minutes before she put the pencil down.

'Done!' she exclaimed.

'Vivian,' I asked softly, 'can you please read it for me? Read slowly and feel it.'

She started reading what she had written.

'I wish to be in a job where I am valued.

'I wish to be comfortable with myself in every relationship that I will be in.

'I wish to have good physical health. I will ensure that I go to the gym regularly.

'I wish that I didn't have to take any medicines. I will be doing my yoga and meditation regularly.

'I wish to keep seeing Dr Pandit for psychotherapy.

'I wish to join a trekking group and go on long treks.

'I wish to own a lot of books and have a small library in my house.

'I wish to learn to dance because I enjoy it. I will join a dancing class.

'I wish to become more religious and attend prayer sessions.

'I wish to finish the translation for *Barom Kagyu*.

'I wish to be better with my investments and finances.

'I wish to have the strength to rebuild myself lovingly and gently, healing with love and light with God's strength.

'I wish to be more social and get to know more people.

'I wish to help people in need.

'I wish to contribute to the community, to the world.

'I wish to travel and get to know people around the world.'

When she looked up from the notepad, she had a glow on her face. She had been to a world of her hidden desires, and that experience seemed to fill her whole being with a lot of positive energy.

When she had walked in, her thoughts were consumed by Kevin's departure from her life. She seemed to have lost every shred of hope for a better life, and by the end of it, she had begun to realise that her life was so much more than Kevin.

I wanted her to be in this state and ended the session.

## 11

It was now more than six months since I had started the therapy sessions with Vivian.

During this period, a lot had happened in Vivian's life, some things due to circumstances beyond her control and others due to her desire to be well. I must admit, she has been one of my more disciplined clients. The law of attraction states that you only get what you desire deeply, and Vivian's thoughts and actions exuded the desire to live the life of her dreams.

She was more in control of herself now. She was still with the same company, and I did not hear from Mr Peter May again, which suggested all was well at work. She seemed to have gotten over Kevin's departure from her life, as she did not speak about him at all. She was always looking ahead, and her perspectives during the book reading sessions suggested that.

It was now time to detach myself from her.

'Vivian, you love children,' I stated in one of the sessions.

'Yes, I do Dr Pandit,' she responded.

'How would you like it if you had a chance to spend a couple of hours with children?' I asked, even though I knew the answer.

'I would love it,' she said, and her expression suggested she meant it.

'I know of a children's home where they take care of children who do not have anyone to care for them. Would you like to spend a couple of hours with them?' I asked.

'Of course, I would like to do it!' she exclaimed.

'You would have heard of the Salvation Army centre.'

Tears welled in her eyes on hearing the name.

'Of course I have heard about it,' she said. 'I have lived there for many years.'

I smiled. 'Why don't you visit them again?' I suggested.

As expected, Vivian had a lot to share when she came for the next session.

'Dr Pandit,' she stated in all excitement, 'you are amazing.'

I smiled as an acknowledgement.

'Thank you for your suggestion,' she said. 'It was so wonderful to be with the kids. I revisited my own childhood. The few hours I spent there filled my heart with gratitude. I was one of them many years ago, and the lovely people over there had given me hope. They had bestowed so much love on me when I did not mean anything to them. The home had supported me in my education. I would be betraying their love if I didn't make something out of my life.'

I smiled upon hearing the response that I had anticipated.

'That's wonderful, Vivian. What do you plan to do?' I enquired.

She replied, 'The centre is doing great work by not only taking care of but supporting the children to build a good life for themselves. The children are so adorable. They shared their dreams with me. I felt so inspired by their positive outlook on life. I spent time with the volunteer team as well. I have offered to conduct book reading sessions at the centre every Friday morning.'

Her enthusiasm was palpable.

I looked deep into her eyes and spoke gently. 'Vivian, you have lived a very different shade of life that I can only imagine. You have lost people who have been close to you at various times. That was how life was meant to be. It's not your fault, and you could not have done anything about it.'

She was listening attentively.

'Look at every difficult situation again from a different perspective. In every moment of tragedy, there was a ray of hope. When your dad met with an accident, the old man gave you hope. When you were at the children's home, the people there gave you hope. When you were all alone, books gave you hope. When the future appeared dark, education gave you hope, and finally, when Kevin moved out of your life, these children have now given you hope.'

She wiped her tears and nodded her head in acknowledgement of what I had said.

I took her hand in mine and said softly, 'Next to *love*, the most important word in the English dictionary is *hope*.'

Beginning the following week, Vivian spent a couple of hours at the centre, reading stories to the children. She found the peace of mind that was missing from her life. For someone who could not share more than a couple of routine tasks when asked how she spent her day, she now had a rather busy-looking calendar. The time spent with the children was bringing much-needed energy and enthusiasm into Vivian's life.

I felt that she was ready for the next step.

'Vivian, I know your days are rather busy, but I suggest one more activity for you,' I told her when she came for her now fortnightly visit to the clinic.

'Dr Pandit, I will do whatever you tell me,' she assured me.

'I want you to visit the Bishan Home for the Mentally Challenged this week,' I suggested. 'Here, they take care of people who are mentally ill and give them a reason to smile.'

And she did that.

'Dr Pandit,' she said when we met after a few weeks, 'you are giving me an opportunity to do so many different things that are bringing me closer to God. I feel so proud of myself now that I am also contributing to society. I got a chance to speak to the lovely people at the home. Most of them are so lonely, as their family members don't come to visit them. But they still keep going. Even with all their challenges, they seem excited with the small joys of life. I reflected on my life not so long ago and realised how small my problems were in comparison to the challenges that these people were facing. I had a big realisation.'

She paused and looked at me.

'It dawned upon me that the challenges in my life were due to my wrong choices. In their case, they do not even have a choice. This is how nature has meant them to be. I realised how I have been wasting this wonderful gift of life that God has given me. I have made a promise to myself ...'

'And what is that?' I enquired.

She continued, 'When I was bidding goodbye, some of them held my hand and did not let go. I decided at that very moment that I am going to devote my life to serve these lovely people.'

I could see tears in her eyes. Unlike the many times these tears had made their appearance, this time, they were tears of joy.

'I am so proud of you, Vivian.' I beamed. 'You have really come a long way. My intention was to show you that we should be grateful for what we have. For all the problems one may be having, there will always be someone else in this world who has bigger problems. Let us thank the Supreme Power for the way we have been created, each with our own unique abilities. Let us express gratitude for every breath we take, and we will see the positivity entering our lives.'

'Dr Pandit,' she said, 'I could sit here and listen to you all day. You are a wonderful therapist. More importantly, you are a wonderful person. I am now beginning to understand how you first motivated me and then reprimanded me when I did not do well, but always continued with the encouragement. Your therapies to help me get over the anxiety attacks, the idea to get me back to my books, and your suggestion to visit to the orphanage and then the Bishan home were all so effective. I cannot thank you enough.'

She came forward and held both my hands in her hands and kissed them. I was touched.

'Vivian, I am so happy to see this real version of you. This is also the moment when I must tell you that you don't need any therapy now.'

'No way!' she exclaimed. 'I need you.'

After some thought, she continued, 'Can I continue to come here at least once a month?'

'You don't need me, Vivian,' I said. 'The world needs you. Your love, your compassion, your energy. You need to fulfil your dream of contributing to society and helping people in need.'

'I want to be like you,' she said. 'I want to help people who are mentally ill and depressed. How can I do that?'

'Becoming a therapist is a long process, and I would not suggest that,' I advised. 'You can, however, do a certification course in therapy. That will give you a basic understanding of how to deal with people who are mentally ill. You can then offer real help to people who need it.'

'I will do that,' she asserted. 'Where do I start?'

I shared some details. I bid her goodbye as a patient but agreed that we would meet once a month and share our experiences with life.

Vivian completed the three-month certification course in therapy. She would share her learnings with me when we would meet. She was a quick learner, and in a short period, she was proficient enough to assist people with mental disorders. I was confident enough to let her assist me with some of my clients who were suffering from mild conditions. She would visit their homes and provide therapy, and I received good feedback for her work.

It's been two years since I first met her, and Vivian is now a confident, independent career woman today. She devotes her time beyond work to many social causes. She has developed a huge network of friends and an impressive list of fans who love her for being there for them. She is still single, although she goes on the occasional date. She has graduated from being my client to an assistant and now to a friend.

When we finished our coffee at the One°15 Marina club, Vivian remarked with a smile, 'I have one more piece of news to share.'

I waited in anticipation.

'I have changed my name,' she said. 'Rather, I have gone back to my original name.'

I gave her a quizzical look.

She shared a piece of information which was never revealed during her sessions with me: 'When the old man brought me to China, he named me Vivian after his own daughter.'

'Oh! And what was your original name?' I asked.

'Fei Hong,' she stated proudly.

'Congratulations!' I exclaimed.

'And do you know what it means?' she asked. 'A swan soaring in the sky.'

'Wow,' I exclaimed.

'And that's exactly what I am going to be now,' she announced excitedly.

As we bid goodbye and were leaving the One°15 Marina club, I gave her a warm hug and whispered in her ear, 'I am proud of you.'

# CHAPTER 5

## CAUSE AND CONSEQUENCE

### 1

'Welcome to *World Sport*. I am Sofia Bussinger.'

The scene was the newsroom of a prominent media house at the Time Warner Center in New York City, and the girl hosting the *World Sport* show that day was Sofia Bussinger. She had joined the media company a year ago and after completing the rigorous induction process was now debuting on *World Sport*. For the millions of people from around the world watching the show, Sofia was the epitome of a dream coming true. The beautiful brunette with deep blue eyes and features to die for was definitely living her dream.

'That's all from the *World of Sport*. Good night.'

As the cameras stopped recording, the entire studio stood up to applaud the newest entrant to their media empire.

The producer, Mr Mark Richards, came forward and shook her hand.

'That was awesome, Sofia,' he exclaimed. 'Welcome to our world.'

'Thank you so much Mark,' a jubilant Sofia replied.

Almost every person in the unit acknowledged that Sofia had indeed done a fabulous job for a first-timer.

That night, as her cab crossed the George Washington Bridge, Sofia looked up at the night sky. The stars brought back flashes of her childhood. As a child, she would spend hours gazing fondly at the stars. Her mother would tell stories of great men and women of this world who died and became twinkling stars. Even from those early years of her life, Sofia always wanted to be in the limelight. She wanted to become a twinkling star.

'Could you please stop the cab?' she suddenly instructed the driver.

The startled driver responded, 'What?'

'Please stop the cab,' she repeated in a louder voice.

'I can't do that, lady,' the now irritated driver retorted. 'We are on the George Washington Bridge.'

She was now screaming, 'I don't care where you are. Just stop the fucking car.'

The driver brought the car to a screeching halt and the bridge was suddenly drowned in a cacophony of horns.

Before he could react, she was out of the cab. She ran to the edge and with a sudden jerk flung herself over the railing into the dark waters of the Hudson River below.

The panic-stricken cab driver made an emergency call from his cell phone.

<h2 style="text-align:center">2</h2>

She opened her eyes and found herself in a strange room. She looked around to see some instruments with blinking lights. She suddenly felt the twitching pain in her left wrist and realised that a needle was inserted there. She was completely blank and could not figure out where she was and what she was doing there. It was a while before a face appeared above her.

'What is this place?' she whispered.

The duty nurse at the Lincoln Hospital spoke in a hushed tone. 'You have been in this hospital since yesterday.'

'Hospital!' she blurted out. 'But … why?'

'You will know,' the lady said and made her way out of the room.

In less than a minute, the door opened, and a police officer walked in.

She was huge and had a commanding presence as she walked to the side of the bed and addressed Sofia in a brusque tone. 'I am Officer Sarah Jones. Would you be able to speak?'

'Huh?' was all Sofia could say, unsure of what was happening.

'What's your name?' the officer asked.

Sofia stared at her blankly and slowly responded nervously, 'Sofia. Sofia Bussinger.'

'You jumped into the Hudson and we had to fish you out, ma'am,' the officer remarked.

'What?' she exclaimed, even more perplexed now.

'Yes, ma'am,' the officer continued. 'And what made you jump into the Hudson?'

'I don't know,' she screamed.

The officer stepped back.

Sofia was hysterical by now. 'Leave me alone,' she screamed, and the tears came out in a flood. 'What am I doing here?'

The nurse rushed back into the room and requested that the officer leave Sofia alone for now.

# 3

Sofia was a good student and did reasonably well in school. It was in high school that she started developing some strange tendencies. She was in grade 12 at a Los Angeles high school, where she met Bill. He was her classmate. A couple of dates later, she was in bed with him. For him, it was a casual fling, but for her, it was so much more than that. The liaison did not last long, and it left her with many emotional scars. A couple of months later, a medical test for an upset stomach revealed that she was pregnant. She was just 16 years old, and this was a bitter shock. The abortion took a toll on her, both physically and mentally, and she started avoiding boys completely. However, it did not last long.

Just a year later, she fell in love with a guy who was much older than her. Emilio was a Spanish hunk, and they met while she was on holiday in Europe. One thing led to another, and she was in bed with him more than a few times. In a couple of months, she became pregnant again. She was 17 and about to enter college. She underwent another abortion and slipped into a state of depression. She needed a shoulder to cry on and a hand to hold for comfort, but Emilio just disappeared. It took her a while to come to grips with herself. She enrolled for a course in media studies at the University of Southern California. She was doing reasonably well in her academics, but her personal life was in shambles. She could not trust anybody, and this behaviour drew people away from her. The frustration led to many bouts of binge drinking. After one such binge night, she ended up in bed with a stranger and sure enough was pregnant for the third time. The doctors advised her against another abortion, as it would leave a permanent scar on her psyche, but as a student away from family, she had no choice. She was a nervous wreck, and it was only her books which helped her still stand on her feet. She secured the third rank in the university, which was no mean feat considering her own state of mind and the pedigree of the institution.

It was no surprise, therefore, that a renowned media house came calling. The break seemed to push her problems to the background, at least briefly. She put her heart and mind into her work and stood out amongst the many new faces who had joined with her. And then Robert Dempsey happened.

Robert had joined the media house about three years prior and had made a mark in a very short time. He was presently part of a team involved in a special assignment. He was the typical well-educated, suave, and to top it off, good-looking man of every girl's dreams. While there were many girls who would do anything to be seen with him, his heart fell for Sofia. The more she tried to avoid him, the more he persisted. It was not long before Sofia's resistance melted, and they were together. For Sofia, the time spent with Robert was the best in her young lifetime. They spent a lot of time together, and with each passing day, Sofia was more head over heels in love with him.

On the career front, she was getting noticed by the people who mattered, for her ideas and for the energy with which she implemented them. And in a fairy-tale moment, she was given the opportunity to host the *World Sport* show. Her joy knew no bounds. Finally, the heavens were conspiring in her favour, and her personal and professional life were falling into place.

And then it happened. The moment she had been waiting for. Her debut was a hit, and she was over the moon with the accolades she received from the unit. She desperately wanted to share the news with the one person whom she loved dearly.

It was 10 p.m., and Sofia knew that Robert would be at his home on Eleventh Avenue, which was just a ten-minute walk from the studio. She had been to his apartment only once in the past, but she trusted her memory and decided to surprise him. She was all excited and couldn't wait to be with Robert and share her experience. She did not have the patience even to wait for the elevator, so she climbed the three flights of stairs. She stopped in her stride as she saw a couple engaged in a passionate kiss just outside Robert's apartment. She waited for a brief moment and was just about to make a move when the couple moved back. Her heart skipped more than a beat as she recognised the man in the dim light of the passage.

It was Robert!

She could not move, and her head went blank. She felt limp and was about to collapse when she took a step back and sat down on the stairway away from their view. She just sat there motionless, staring at the dark wall in front of her for a long time. From the heights of euphoria just some moments ago, she had been thrown into the depths of despair.

Suddenly, she stood up and ran down the stairway. Once out, she hailed a cab and instructed the driver to just drive. Her head was reeling with the plethora of emotions that had engulfed her during the past couple of hours. So many thoughts were racing through her head, and nothing made any sense to her except one.

'Drive through the George Washington Bridge,' she instructed the driver.

The driver looked at her from the rear-view mirror and took the turn which would take them to the George Washington bridge.

## 4

The police officer continued to grill her.

'Where do you live?'

'Where do you work?'

'Where is your family?'

And 'Why did you jump in the Hudson River?'

With every answer, her bitterness grew, and the tears wouldn't stop. She almost cried herself into a state of unconsciousness.

The sound of someone calling out her name woke her up. She slowly opened her eyes to see a couple of faces looking down on her. She looked around and realised she was still in the hospital bed.

'Welcome back,' the lady said. 'I am Dr Su Barker.'

She seemed so much more humane than the police officer who had interrogated her.

'I understand your name is Sofia Bussinger,' she remarked.

Sofia nodded.

'Do you have anyone from your close family here?' she asked.

'No, I live alone,' Sofia replied.

'OK, I want you to first have some orange juice and then take some rest. We will give you some food after some time so that you regain your strength.'

She looked at the nurse. 'I don't want anyone to come and meet her without my permission.'

The next morning, Sofia woke up feeling so much better. She buzzed the nurse who helped her to the toilet. She had a light breakfast of toast and butter.

'I see you are up already,' Dr Su Barker walked into the room with her trademark exuberance.

'Yes, Doctor.' Sofia smiled. 'I feel much better today.'

The doctor came and sat next to Sofia and held her hand.

'Do you have a boyfriend?' she asked.

Sofia was taken aback by the question.

'I … I …' she fumbled for an answer.

'Sorry to have broached this subject,' the doctor said, 'but it was necessary in this situation.'

Sofia did not answer.

Dr Su Barker held her hand even more tightly and spoke.

'Sofia, you are pregnant.'

The statement was like a bolt from the blue. She could not believe her ears. How could this happen? How could this happen again?

Feeling her hands go numb, the doctor gently stroked Sofia's hair.

'Sofia, do you know who the father is?' she asked softly.

Sofia nodded.

'Do you want to call him?' she asked.

Sofia turned her head and sunk her head in the pillow. She was crying hysterically. So many thoughts were going through her head, but nothing seemed to make sense.

The doctor waited patiently and when the tears stopped, she asked another question.

'Do you want the baby?'

Sofia did not respond but the doctor could hear her intermittent sniffs.

'Sofia,' the doctor said, 'I know this is a very difficult time for you. But it is also important that you make a decision on the baby soon. We cannot abort the foetus after a couple of weeks.'

She continued, 'I will leave you now. I will advise the nurse to take you out for a walk. You definitely need some fresh air.'

The room was silent again.

Sofia remained in the curled-up position on the bed wondering where her life was heading. It was just a couple of days ago when she was on top of the world. And now she was back to her familiar feeling of despondency. It was only a matter of time before her office would know about her secrets.

She needed to talk to someone, someone with whom she could open her heart and she made the call.

'Mumma,' she screamed when her phone was answered.

'Baby!' her mother exclaimed. 'What happened, dear?'

'I am missing you, Mumma,' she cried.

Her mother was worried now.

'My baby,' she said softly, 'please calm down and tell me what happened. I am always here for you.'

Her tirade continued, 'Mumma, I want to come to you. I want you to just hold me.'

Her mother spoke a little more sternly. 'Listen to me. Just calm down … just calm down.' She kept repeating it until she was sure that Sofia had indeed calmed down.

'Mumma, my life is in a mess,' she blurted out.

'My baby,' her mummy muttered lovingly, 'whatever problem you are in, we can find a way out.'

Sofia continued to speak, 'Every time I feel things are getting better, it only becomes even worse than what it was before. I want to be with you.'

'Then why don't you come? It been more than a year that you have come home anyway,' her mother suggested.

Just hearing those words made Sofia feel so much better.

'Even before you do that, I want you to speak to someone whom I know can help you sort out your life,' her mother continued.

Sofia was listening.

'I want you to call Dr Preeti Pandit. She is a psychotherapist in Singapore,' her mother said.

They continued talking for some time.

Sofia did feel a little better after the call. However, she had never felt as lonely as she was feeling at that moment. Alone in the cold hospital room, with only the beeping sound of the electrocardiogram for company, she felt really alone. She could just sit there and not do anything about it, or she could take charge of her life. She decided to do the latter.

# 5

It was a hot day in Singapore, and the humidity was at its peak. I always keep a stock of electrolytes in my clinic just for days like these. I started sipping the cool drink from a tetra pack when the intercom buzzed. It was Sandra asking me to answer the phone.

'Am I speaking to Dr Preeti Pandit?' the lady asked.

'Yes, I am Dr Preeti Pandit,' I responded.

'Hope I am not disturbing you at this hour?' she enquired politely.

'Not at all,' I said. 'May I know who is speaking?'

'My name is Sofia Bussinger,' the lady stated. 'I got your reference from my mother, Emma Bussinger. She said that she knows you well.'

I jogged my memory and replied, 'Of course I know her.'

'I need some help,' she said, 'and Mumma said that you are the best person for that.'

'Sofia,' I said, 'I would definitely help if it is in my capacity.'

'My life is a mess,' she remarked. 'Every day I feel that I am turning a corner, but I seem to come back to where I was—and most times even worse.'

'I can help you Sofia,' I said. 'We would need to meet so that I hear your complete story. When can you come?'

'I live in New York,' she said. 'Can't we talk on the phone?'

That was a surprise. I do get international calls from my clients, but this was the first time someone was calling from America to become one.

'No, dear,' I confirmed. 'I don't do psychotherapy over long distance.'

She seemed to be thinking as the phone went silent.

'OK,' she said, 'I will come and meet you. Give me a few days, and I will confirm the date.'

That seemed strange. Why would someone travel from New York to Singapore to meet me?

I replayed the call in my head and said to myself, 'Hmmm … Emma's daughter.'

On an impulse, I reached for my diary and referred to my notes on Emma.

# 6

To have a glimpse of heaven on earth, all one needs to do is visit Switzerland. The country has been blessed with so much of natural beauty that one can actually get bored with it. God seems to have employed His master craftsman to design this place, its weather, and its people. Time seems to stand still in this beautiful country.

I was in Switzerland for some work and was staying at a bed and breakfast in Lucerne. Every morning, after a sumptuous breakfast, I would walk along the streets of this lovely city. I would spend some time on the Chapel Bridge, the iconic winding bridge lined with art, and then sit and admire the famous sculpture of the Lion Monument. The Swiss Museum of Transport was another attraction I had visited a couple of times. Once my work was done by early afternoon, I would pack some sandwiches and head for the riverside park. Sitting by the river with a book in hand was like finding paradise.

This was my routine for the past three days that I was here, and I estimated my sojourn to last for another week.

I would sit by the river and watch the people around me. Every day, there would be a few singletons sitting on their portable chairs with a book in hand. There would be a few couples sharing some intimate moments and some families with children engaged in a game. There was one thing which seemed common among every person I had seen ever since I arrived here. Everyone seemed so happy and why wouldn't they be? They were literally living in the happiest country in the world.

That was until my eyes fell on her.

In her white dress, she was like the swan among a flock of ducks. Her long hair was gently blowing in the breeze. In spite of the general quietude around her, she was serenity personified. The skin on her face and hands were glowing in the mild afternoon sun, and her eyes seemed to be reflecting the blue of Lake Lucerne. In fact, her beauty seemed to enhance the picturesque surroundings. What stood out though was her forlorn appearance. A first look suggested she was lost in thought, but a keener eye could sense she was morose.

The realisation dawned upon me after a few minutes that I had been staring at her. I just couldn't take my eyes off her, such was her beauty. I forced myself to turn my head away from her and walked away. It should have been the last glimpse of her, but fate had other plans.

The next day, there she was again. In her yellow dress, she seemed even more beautiful. Except for the dress, everything about the scene was exactly the same as yesterday.

I could not hold back my curiosity any longer, and I walked towards her and sat down on the grass just a few feet away.

'A lovely afternoon,' I said to no one in particular.

The object of my comment, however, did not respond.

I waited for some time and tried again. This time I was more direct.

'This is such a wonderful place. Do you come here often?' I directly addressed her.

She turned her head and a faint smile appeared on her lips.

'Yes, it's a beautiful place,' she replied.

Her accent suggested she was not European.

Having established contact, I continued, 'My name is Preeti, and I am from Singapore.'

She replied softly.

'My name is Emma. I am from Bali.'

*That explains the accent*, I thought.

'Bali is a lovely place,' I said. 'I have been there on holiday once. Are you here on holiday?'

The question seemed to lull her into silence. Maybe it was too personal. Her expressions changed and her gaze shifted away from me.

I did not speak, waiting for her to continue the conversation, but it never happened.

After a few minutes of continued silence, I wished her goodbye and left.

My work in Singapore finished much earlier than I had planned, and I rescheduled my travel plans. I still had a day to spare and decided to soak in some of the sunshine around the lakefront.

I walked on the narrow path close to the pristine waters of the lake deep in my own thoughts, when I heard someone calling, 'Excuse me, ma'am.'

I turned back and there she was, as beautiful as ever, in a frock filled with floral designs. Her hair was tied in a ponytail, and she had a yellow flower pinned on it. Standing there, Emma looked like an angel who had descended from the heavens. Her slightly plump figure gave her a motherly touch.

I waited for her to reach me.

'Dear lady,' she said in between her deep breaths, 'I am very sorry about yesterday.'

I smiled at her. 'You don't have to worry,' I said calmly. 'If anyone has to be sorry, it should be me. I had intruded into your privacy.'

'No, no,' she said quickly, 'you are a kind person, and I just ignored you.'

I did not respond, wanting to end that line of conversation.

'Would you have coffee with me?' she requested.

I did not have any other plans for that evening, and I agreed.

'It's silly of me,' she confessed sheepishly. 'I even forgot your name.'

'It's Dr Preeti Pandit,' I replied.

'And I am Emma,' she said and asked, 'Can I call you Dr Preeti?'

'Yes, you can,' I confirmed.

The lakefront has several small cafes, which serve pastries, chocolate, and coffee.

We settled down in a comfortable corner of one such café and ordered a pastry and coffee.

'I don't know why,' Emma said, 'when you approached me yesterday, I felt there was something about you which made me feel like talking to you. But I was not sure if I should. What's the point of doing it?'

'Emma, let me tell you more about myself,' I suggested with a smile. 'That may help you make a decision.'

She was listening attentively.

'I am a therapist,' I said, 'and I work with people who are trying to find answers to questions about life. I even help people to understand what those questions should be. Let me share something with you. When I saw you for the first time a couple of days ago, your beauty caught my eye, but what also struck me was the melancholy in your eyes and gloom around you. A trained eye could sense that something was wrong. I made conversation with you to see if I could help.'

She almost leapt up from her chair, and the excitement in her voice was palpable.

'I can't believe it,' she exclaimed. 'I was searching for some answers, and it looks like God has sent you to help me find them.'

'Maybe,' I said.

She leaned forward and held my hand. 'Would you help me, Dr Preeti?' she asked with complete sincerity.

'Of course I will,' I affirmed, and then the thought struck me: *We need to sort a few things before we can get going.*

'Please, Dr Preeti, I need your help,' she pleaded.

'Please listen to me,' I said. 'I go back to Singapore tomorrow. I do speak to my clients over the phone and offer some advice from time to time, but I do not practise or recommend long-distance therapy.'

Emma thought about it, but not for long.

'I will be going back to Bali in a few weeks,' Emma explained, 'and I am ready to come to Singapore for a few days whenever you suggest.'

She seemed very keen to make this happen.

'In that case, let's begin,' I remarked.

And she shared her story.

# 7

Emma was born in Bali to Indonesian parents. Her father was a tourist guide and would earn enough to take care of his family of five, which included his wife, Emma, and her two sisters. Emma's mother had an artistic trait in her and would do a lot of sketching in her spare time. Many of her sketches were that of the jewellery worn by tourists visiting the island, but some would also be from her own imagination. The designs would include a lot of materials found locally like different shapes and sizes of seashells, stones, and gems.

Emma developed a liking for crafts, and from a young age, she started crafting the jewellery based on her mother's designs. Her passion and attention to detail ensured that her creations started getting appreciated by people. This encouraged Emma to convince her father to invest in a stall at the Pasar Badung market, an open-air market frequented by tourists. Her father would get tourists to her stall, and it did not take too long for her designs to find buyers. Very soon, she had to employ a couple of girls who could make the jewellery for her. What started as a hobby soon turned into a good business. Just when life was looking good, tragedy struck. Her mother passed away due to a prolonged illness, and as the eldest child, Emma had to don the role of a mother for her two younger siblings. Emma's life now alternated between the chores at home and needs of the business.

It was the month of December, and tourists were slowly trickling in for the festive season ahead. Bali was lit up, and very soon, there would be many parties and events organised across the island. The Pasar Badung market was a twenty-four-hour market, and during the peak season, it would be teeming with tourists. Like every year, Emma would look forward to this time of the year, when her business was at its peak. For her, the tourists from all over the world were just customers who appreciated her work of art. They were just unknown faces but this year one of those faces belonged to David.

David was a Swiss native and was visiting Bali for the first time. He happened to visit the Pasar Badung market that evening, and while browsing through the variety of items on display, his eyes fell on Emma. He was enamoured by her beauty. He watched her from a distance as she showed her jewellery to customers. He couldn't take his eyes off her long hair blowing in the light breeze (and her repeated attempts to move it away from her eyes); her dazzling smile, which seemed to light up her shop; her beautiful face, which was as radiant as the moon above her; and those lovely blue eyes, which seemed to sparkle even from this distance.

For the next few days, he did not bother going around Bali. He would wait for the afternoon and then perch himself at a spot which was some distance away from Emma's store but close enough for him to have an uninterrupted view. With his departure date from Bali approaching, he had to make an approach.

David was not the quintessential handsome man. In fact, he was far from it. At 35, he was slightly bald and had a generous rather than an athletic body. But what he had in abundance was a pleasant personality, the ability to warm up to people, and the gift of speech. It did not take too long for him to win over Emma's heart. In the three days that they established contact, Emma saw a charming, warm, and kind person in him and was drawn to him. They remained in touch even when David went back home.

Within six months, David was back in Bali, and this time, he stayed in the room at Emma's parents' home, which was up for rent. This gave them an opportunity to spend more time with each other, and they developed a more intimate relationship. Emma was only twenty-four, but the difference in age did not matter to her. For Emma, it was like a lovely dream she was living, and she did not want to wake up. Her fondness for David was growing with every passing day, and it reached a crescendo when, one night, while they were at the beach on a full moon night, David went down on his knees and proposed to her.

Her heart skipped a beat. Everything was happening so fast. Her heart wanted to say yes and be with David for the rest of her life, and her mind wanted her to consider the implications.

Well, her heart won the one-sided contest.

With David back in Switzerland, she spent the next few months convincing her family and dreaming about the good life. Everything seemed to fall in place, and they decided to get married when David would visit Bali in a few months.

The fairy-tale romance between a beautiful Balinese lady and a charming Swiss man culminated in a grand wedding on the beaches of Bali.

Their honeymoon extended for many months. David would fly down to Bali every six months and spend a few weeks. He had a flourishing restaurant business in Zurich, and he couldn't be away from it for too long. He liked Emma's jewellery designs and started carrying them back home. He used a corner of his restaurant to display her creations and very soon found a receptive audience. Their relationship also had a positive impact on Emma's business.

After one of his trips to Bali, he took her back to Switzerland. They continued their honeymoon in the snow-capped Alps. They visited other parts of Europe and spent a few days visiting the tourist attractions there. Back home in Bali, a radiant Emma continued to live her dream and it got even better with the realisation that she was pregnant. Their liaison gave birth to a beautiful girl whom she would lovingly call 'Dewi' (the goddess), and in a couple of years, they had a handsome boy who she proudly called 'Intan' (diamond). Emma and the children lived in Bali, and David would visit them twice in a year and ensured that he made up for the time in between.

It was indeed a fairy tale, which was destined to end in 'they all lived happily ever after ...'

But then ... this was real life.

# 8

The Balinese are traditional people and hold family values and culture in high esteem. Emma and her children lived with her father and her two sisters in their big house. Her father was away from home most of the time, since his work required a lot of travel, and the children never got the opportunity to get pampered by their grandparents. Seeing the other children around them, the obvious question to their father when he came visiting was 'Papa, when can we meet our grandparents?'

During all their years of marriage, Emma had known about David's parents living in Switzerland and she even expressed the desire to meet them. While David did not refuse, he never took the initiative to make the meeting happen either. For someone who was smitten by David, Emma did not find any reason to question this behaviour.

Now that his children were asking this question, and toddlers can be very persistent, David let go of whatever inhibitions he harboured and promised to take them to Switzerland the next time he would be returning from Bali. And they did not let him forget his promise. Every time he would call Emma from Switzerland and speak to them, this question came up every time. Very soon, Emma also joined the chorus and with David's help planned the trip to Switzerland with the specific intention of meeting her parents-in-law.

## 9

Appenzell is a small village in the Swiss Alps. Surrounded by the natural beauty of the Alps, the traditional architecture and colourful facades of Appenzell's main square and street draw visitors to its centre year after year. It is also the home to an impressive castle, Catholic church, and mural-covered town hall. Less than 100 km from Zurich, Appenzell was the home of David's family for generations. They still lived in a palatial home on the mountains. The house is almost undetectable, as it is nestled right into the mountains. Set below ground, the concrete structure features a wide oval opening that one arrives at via a set of stones steps embedded in the steep incline. At the top of the stairs, a central patio is surrounded by a wide-spanning facade formed of large window openings, which provide luminous reflections of the alpine vista on the opposite side of the narrow valley. A huge living room with a fireplace and life-size paintings on its walls completed the traditional look. David's ancestors had close links with the royal family, which resulted in them amassing a lot of wealth which was enough to feed a few generations. And it showed.

Emma and the children accompanied David to Zurich and from there they embarked on the journey by road to their ancestral home.

They were greeted by David's mother when they reached their home. She was a plump woman with golden hair and a round, chubby face, which seemed to always smile. She wore a light blue frock with frills, and with her short stature, she seemed like a teddy bear.

'Welcome to Appenzell,' David's mother greeted Emma warmly as she stepped out of the car.

'Thank you so much,' Emma responded with a smile and a shake of her hand.

'And where are my grandchildren?' she asked as she looked inside the car.

The toddlers stepped out to be greeted with a warm hug from their grandmother.

'And what are your names?' she asked lovingly.

'My name is Dewi, and his name is Intan,' the girl answered.

Emma wanted to share their real names, but she decided to do it sometime later.

The warm welcome made the children immediately connect with their grandmother, and they had no reservations about holding on to her hand as she led them into the house.

David held Emma's hand as they followed. She was dumbfounded by the grandiose of the place. Emma's house in Bali was also big, but in comparison to this villa, it now seemed tiny. A maid took care of their luggage as they made their way into the main living room. Here, they met David's father.

He was a staid-looking gentleman, quite unlike his extrovert son. His grey moustache and beard added to his grave look. He wore a three-piece suit and a typical Swiss hat. A cigar in his lips complemented the royal appearance.

David greeted him with a hug and introduced the new arrivals.

'Pa, she is Emma,' he said, gesturing towards Emma.

'And here are your grandchildren Dewi and Intan,' David's mother interjected in all excitement.

'Hello,' David's father responded with just the hint of a smile.

Sensing Emma's discomfort, David stepped in to end the silence.

'You may be tired after the long journey,' he said loudly and added with a smirk, 'At least I am.'

'Yes, my dearies, it's time for some rest,' his mother added as she addressed the children.

The next few days were spent in exploring the village, taking long walks along the narrow lanes, browsing through stuff at the local market, and trekking up the hills. The children were having a wonderful time, with their grandmother pampering them with delicacies every hour of the day. Emma was happy to be with David and his family. But something was bothering her. While David's mother had accepted her children as family, she had hardly spent quality time with Emma. David's father hardly spoke to anyone in the house, so it did not matter that there had been no conversation with him at all. More importantly, David also seemed a bit tense and was not in his usual carefree self. She dismissed the thought quickly and decided to take the initiative in building the relationship with her parents-in-laws.

## 10

It was a lovely June morning in Appenzell. The sun was out in its full glory, and the bright light reflected off the ice-covered peaks of the Alps, making the place seem even brighter. Emma woke up and realised that David was not around. She lay in bed and gazed admiringly at the mountains through the huge window. The lovely weather and the heavenly scenery made her feel really happy. She quickly dressed and walked downstairs. David was about to leave the house when he saw her.

'Good morning, my darling,' he said and came forward to take her in his arms. 'I did not want to disturb your beauty sleep, so I did not wake you up.'

'Good morning, my dear,' Emma responded with a tight embrace.

David continued, 'I have to meet someone in Zurich. I will be back by evening. I leave you in the good care of my mother.' He winked as he said that.

Very soon, his mother too seemed ready to step out of the house. 'I am going to the local market to buy some fresh bread and cake,' she declared, and the two children followed her gleefully.

Emma realised that she would be alone with David's father.

*Maybe this is a good time to have a conversation with him,* she thought.

She looked around and found him in the study, engrossed in a book. She tiptoed close to him and whispered, 'I am very sorry to disturb you. It's just that we have been here for a few days and I never had an opportunity to know you. Is this a good time?'

David's father looked up from the book.

He closed the book and walked towards the sofa under the window. He sat down and gestured Emma to join him there.

'Hope you are being taken care of by everyone?' he asked in a deep-throated voice.

'Oh, yes!' she exclaimed, glad that he had acceded to her request. 'David calls you Pa. Can I call you that as well?'

He nodded.

She now realised that in her eagerness, she had not really prepared for this conversation. She was searching for the right words when he spoke.

'There is a lot of history to this place,' he said slowly. 'This house is more than 150 years old and dates back to the eighteenth century. He went on to share details of their ancestry and their links with the Landenberg family of nobles.'

He had probably compensated for the silence of the past few days with his long narration. In his deep voice, the history seemed so much more dramatic, and Emma was glad that she had gathered the courage to come forward and have this conversation.

'That's wonderful, Pa,' she said excitedly. 'Thank you so much for sharing it with me.'

He asked Emma about her family in Bali. He seemed well read since he had a few things to say about Bali and its history.

Just as the conversation seemed to get interesting, he very abruptly fell silent as if in deep thought. She was wondering if she had said something inappropriate when he spoke again. His deep-throated voice made his words seem grave.

'I have been wanting to tell you something,' he said, 'and I have been pondering over it since the day you came here. You are a lovely lady, and you seem to have a lovely family back home in Bali. It would be incorrect on my part if I don't share some things with you.'

Emma's emotions changed to that of nervous anticipation on hearing these words.

*What does he want to share with me?* she thought.

She waited with bated breath for her father-in-law to continue.

'I am not sure if David has ever mentioned this to you,' he wondered loudly.

'Mentioned what, Pa?' Emma almost pleaded.

After a moment of silence, he stated, 'That he is already married.'

Emma was not sure whether she heard him right.

'What did you say, Pa?' she enquired.

'Emma,' he clarified, 'David was married before he met you. His wife, Laura, lives with us. Presently, she is in England visiting her family.'

The silence that followed was deafening. She covered her ears with her hands to drown out the noise, but it only grew louder. She felt dizzy and collapsed on the sofa.

She opened her eyes to see the maid with a glass of water. The magnitude of her father-in-law's statement finally hit her, and she burst into tears. They were tears of despair and disbelief. How could this be happening?

'I am sorry that I had to put you in this situation,' David's father apologised when he felt she had regained some control, 'but I had to share this information with you.'

Her tears were still coming in a flood and she wailed, 'Why did he marry me if he was already married? How could you allow him to do that?'

Emma had always been demure, and it was the business which gave her the confidence to face the world. She had never been assertive, and even today, she would take a lot of effort to convince her customers to buy her wares at a price that she wanted. She was averse to conflicts of any kind and would either veer away from them or quickly arrive at a compromise. This was the Emma who had been forced into this complex situation.

David's father was his usual staid self as she bared her emotions in front of him.

'David did tell us about his love for you and his intention to marry you,' he confessed. 'We were completely opposed to the idea and discouraged him rather vehemently, but he still went ahead. His mother and I have not been on good terms with him since then. However, when he broke the news of your child coming into this world, his mother's heart changed. She had yearned to become a grandmother and hold her grandchildren in her arms, something Laura could not give her.'

'And what about Laura?' Emma asked, suddenly realising that there was another person in the equation now.

'She is unaware of your existence,' David's father replied. 'She believes that David needs to travel to Bali on business and will be away for some months in the year.'

'That is so unfair,' she sobbed. 'How could David do this to both of us?'

The avalanche of tears started again and continued for a while.

'I cannot forgive him for this,' she declared, 'and I cannot forgive all of you for this as well. You could have prevented it, but you did not. So many lives have been affected because of you.'

She picked up her dishevelled self and rushed to her room upstairs.

*I cannot stay here any longer*, she thought on the way.

Her mind was racing with possibilities. What would happen to her marriage? Does it even qualify to be a marriage? What about her children? Do they even have a legal status?

She locked herself in the bedroom and cried the entire afternoon.

The knock on the door brought her back to the present. She wiped her tears and opened the door. It was David.

'Hi, darling. How was your day? I am sure you missed me, but I missed you more,' he greeted her with a chuckle and proceeded to take her in his arms.

Emma couldn't hold back her tears and started wailing. She held onto him tightly, and her hands pulled his shirt from the collar.

'Hey,' he muttered softly and ran his fingers through her hair. 'What's the matter?'

She ignored his question and continued to cry loudly. He realised that something was seriously wrong. He held her hands and pushed her slightly away from him so he could see her.

'Emma, my dear,' he said. 'What's the matter?'

'How could you do this to me David?' she bawled.

'What are you talking about Emma?' he asked now with a hint of concern.

In between her sobs, she proclaimed loudly, 'I know about Laura.'

It was David's turn to be speechless.

'What?' he gasped.

'I know about Laura and that she is your wife,' she bellowed. 'In fact, she was your wife even before you met me. How could you do this to me?'

David was dumbfounded. He realised that the truth was out in the open now.

Her tears had turned to anger now.

'Now I realise why you were reluctant to bring me home,' she continued. 'All along, you were betraying me with your bloody lies.'

David stepped forward and held her arms.

'Emma,' he said, 'I want you to listen to me. I really, really love you, and I have loved you since the time I first saw you in Bali.'

'Stop it, David,' she screamed. 'Don't keep lying to me.'

'I am not lying Emma,' he said gently at first and then a little more sternly, 'I am not lying. I fell in love with you when I first saw you in Bali, but I knew it was wrong. When I came back home, I couldn't sleep. I swear to you, Emma, those were some of the most difficult days of my life. I have a good relationship with Laura, but I don't love her. I have never loved anyone the way I felt about you. During those difficult days, I made my decision. I wanted to be with you, make love to you, take care of you, and spend the rest of my life with you. Please tell me, have I ever let you down in all these years?'

He was right. Up until the moment his father revealed the truth, there was no reason for her to complain. David had treated her as a companion and kept her and her family happy.

She continued to sob and did not speak.

'Emma, please believe me. I love you more than anything else in this world. Our children mean so much to me. We can still make this work.'

'How can it work, David?' she finally spoke. 'How can it work when I know that you have a wife who lives with you here? How can it work when I don't even know what my legal status is? And what about our children?'

'They need not know anything Emma,' he responded calmly. 'Things can continue the way it has been over these seven years. We were all happy, and we can all continue to be happy.'

'This may be very easy for you to say, David,' she confessed. 'But this is over for me. Please book me and the children on a flight to Bali today. Let me move out of your life and leave you with your legal wife. I know it will be difficult for me, but I will manage.'

'Emma, please don't do anything in haste,' he pleaded. 'I know all this may seem like I have been unfair with you, but that's not the case. Even when I am here, my heart is with you.'

She interrupted him, 'Then why don't you divorce her and come to Bali with me?'

'I wish I could do that,' he admitted slowly.

Her tone was slowly changing to defiance.

'If you really love me, what is stopping you from leaving her and coming with me?' she asked in anger.

'Emma, it's not that easy,' he explained. 'Laura's family and ours go back a long way. Our families have a rich tradition, and the people in this village and beyond look up to us. Divorce may be more acceptable to the world today, but for this conservative village folks and for our families, it is unthinkable.'

She could not believe her ears.

'Marrying another person when you already have a wife is fine, but divorcing someone you don't love is looked down upon. What kind of a tradition is this?'

'Emma, all this is way too complicated,' he explained. 'I know it a huge shock for you, and why not? But let me say this again. I love you more than anything else in this world, and I will continue to do so. All I request you is to look at this situation calmly and then decide.'

She remained silent.

He continued, 'I will book your tickets to Bali, since it will not be appropriate for you to stay here now. Think this through. We can continue to live happily the way we were living until now. Also, Laura cannot bear any children, so you need not worry about Dewi and Intan.'

Against the wishes of David, his mother who had grown really fond of her grandchildren and did not want to part with them, the children themselves who were finally getting the love from their grandparents, Emma and the children took the next flight out of Zurich.

Through the flight and after coming back home to Bali, she remained deep in thought. What should she do now? Everything David said about his love for her was true, but she couldn't remove Laura from her mind. She could never accept the fact that her husband, the person she loved so much, was married to someone else and was also having a physical relationship with her. True to her personality, she could not and did not take any assertive steps and just let the issue linger on.

She would not show her emotions to her children and the rest of the family but would cry in her room through the night.

She would tell stories to Dewi and Intan of people who had achieved success in their lives and urge them to work hard to achieve their dreams. She neglected her business and her staff left her for better work. She would hardly have any food and refused to go out and meet anyone. She was in a state of severe depression. She did not share any details with her family, and they attributed this behaviour to a possible fight between husband and wife.

## 11

It was more than three months since Emma returned from Appenzell. David had called her almost every day since then, but she would refuse to talk to him, and even if she did, she would only respond in monosyllables. David would speak to her sisters and enquire about her health and share his concern for her.

On that day, the phone rang. Emma's sister, Elena, answered and was greeted by a pleasant voice.

'Hello, dear. How are you doing today?'

Elena did not recognise the voice and asked in her local language, 'Who is speaking?'

'Sorry, dear,' the lady remarked. 'I cannot understand that language.'

Elena quickly changed to English. 'Who is speaking?'

'I am David's mother here,' the lady revealed. 'I would like to speak to Emma.'

'Oh, nice to speak to you, ma'am,' Elena responded apologetically. 'Let me call Emma.'

On Elena's insistence, Emma answered the phone.

'Hello,' she said rather coldly.

'Hello, Emma,' David's mother greeted her. 'How are you doing?'

'I am good,' Emma answered without bothering to reciprocate.

David's mother came to the point.

'Whatever has happened is unfortunate,' she said. 'We have to see what is good for everyone involved. We accept your relationship with David and will ensure that you get all the respect and the rights accorded to a wife. Your children will be David's heirs. What more would you want?'

'All these things don't matter when your love is divided,' Emma said with more than a tinge of sarcasm.

David's mother responded, 'Emma, I agree that love is important. But then, love cannot give you the luxuries of life. Love cannot guarantee the highest level of education for your children. All that can be yours. Nothing needs to change between you and David. Nothing will change between David and Laura.'

Emma did not respond.

'I want to spend more time with my grandchildren. And only you can make that happen. However strained your relationship with David is, it should not get in the way of a grandmother's love for her grandchildren.'

Emma listened.

'Emma, I am sending three tickets for your trip to Zurich. You are welcome to stay with us. If you feel otherwise, you can stay at our house at Lucerne. Your children can stay in Appenzell.'

A question crossed Emma's mind.

'What about Laura?' she asked.

'Laura has no issues with this arrangement,' David's mother answered.

If what David's mother said was true, Emma realised that she was the only person who was unhappy with the situation in hand. Everyone seemed to have accepted it, willingly or otherwise.

Dewi and Intan had loved their stay in David's villa, and there had not been one day since they had come back when they did not talk about going back there. Was it right for her to deprive her children of their grandmother's love and the moments of fun? She had not made a decision on her relationship with David yet, so the offer of staying at Lucerne made sense.

After a lot of internal deliberations, she decided to accept the offer and travel to Appenzell.

And it was on this trip that she met me.

## 12

'What is the question that you want to be answered?' I asked Emma after she had finished narrating her story.

Emma seemed crestfallen as she had lived those bittersweet moments of her life while narrating them to me. We had been sitting in the cafe for more than an hour, and I realised that it was time for me to leave and get ready for my return journey the next day.

'There is a lot going on in your life Emma,' I said softly and then asked again 'Among all the confusion, what is the question that is uppermost in your mind?'

It seemed a straightforward question, but in many cases, we don't find the solution to a problem because we are not able to define the problem in the first place.

'I am confused,' Emma confessed. 'I am torn between my own identity and the bond between a grandmother and grandchildren.'

'Emma, I have heard you,' I said. 'A few sessions of therapy will help, but the question is would you want those sessions? If yes, then I am sure we can find a way.'

'I have never been this depressed in my entire life,' Emma shared. 'I think life has no meaning, and I am only living it for my children. I have no interest in my business or in any relationships.'

'What do you want to do about it?' I asked.

She thought about it and replied, 'I want to have the sessions with you. From the time I met you, I feel a certain comfort level. I have not shared the details of my life with anyone, including my own sisters. But something made me open up to you. I feel you can help me find the answers I am looking for.'

'I am flying back to Singapore tomorrow,' I said. 'Here is my business card. Please call me when you are back in Bali.'

She took the card and glanced at the details. She then held my hand and said, 'I trust you to help me, Dr Preeti.'

I held on to her hand and looked in her eyes. I could see the sincerity in them.

'I will help you, Emma,' I said. 'I definitely will.'


I received the phone call in less than a week. Emma was calling not from Bali but from Switzerland.

'Hello, Dr Preeti,' she announced. 'I am coming to Singapore en route to Bali.'

'When is that?' I asked quickly opening my diary to check my dates.

'It will be the Monday after the coming week,' she replied. 'And I will be there for a week. I would like to meet you every day during that week.

I checked my dates and most days of that week looked busy. *I would have to reschedule some of my appointments*, I thought.

'OK,' I said, 'and where would you be staying?'

Once you confirm, I will be booking into a bed and breakfast accommodation close to your clinic.

'Please go ahead with your plans,' I said and blocked the dates in my diary.

## 13

'What should I do? Should I resign myself to the situation or should I end my relationship with David?' was her question when she came to meet me in Singapore.

She seemed more in control of herself, but there were visible signs of her negative state of mind. The dark circles around her eyes were more visible with her fair skin.

'Are there other options beyond what you have just stated?' I asked, wanting her to consider all the possibilities.

'Well, I could force David to divorce Laura and come and live with me,' she said after some thought.

'Yes, that's an option as well,' I stated. 'What other options can you think of?'

'David's mother may want to keep the children with her, which I will not allow,' she said defiantly.

'Of course, you will not allow that,' I said, 'but that's also a possibility.'

She thought for some more time and declared, 'Those are the options I can think of.'

'What about the option of you accepting the situation wholeheartedly,' I quizzed, 'and the option of David living with you without divorcing his wife?'

'Both are impossible,' she stated without even considering them.

'Your mind has blocked out many such options because you have labelled them as impossible,' I explained, 'but they are possibilities even if the chances are very remote.'

She listened intently.

'Who are the people that you are concerned about in this situation?' I asked.

'My children', she stated, 'and of course me.'

'Who else?' I asked.

'There are others, but whatever decision I take may not affect them,' she said.

'That may be true, but who are they?' I persisted.

'David, my father and sisters, David's parents, Laura. I guess that's it,' she declared.

'And if you were allowed to decide your fate without any constraints, what would that be?'

This question made her really think. She had never gone beyond the two options that she thought existed. After a lot of internal deliberations, she confessed, 'I would want David to come and live with me after divorcing Laura.'

'And whom would this affect?' I probed.

'Well, it would definitely affect Laura,' she opined, 'and it would affect his parents and their reputation.'

'And does this worry you?' I probed further.

As she was searching for an answer, the realisation dawned upon her that she did not want to hurt Laura, as she was not at fault in this entire drama that had unfolded. She did not want to hurt his parents and their reputation since they have been good with her children. And she did not want to hurt David.

'Now do you realise why you have not been able to come to a decision?' I asked.

For the rest of the session and for the next few days, my role was to disconnect herself as a person from the situation in hand and then look at it from all perspectives. This would help her to take a decision which would be the right one for her.

As a therapist, I would not want to recommend any course of action. Who am I to say what is right and what is wrong for

Emma? Nothing is black and white in this world. It becomes so when we disregard possibilities without due consideration.

After four days of intense questioning and introspections, she had arrived at her decision.

'I will accept my current situation since it is the best option for me and for everyone who matters to me. I will let the children spend time with their grandparents from time to time. I would like David to visit me periodically in his capacity as the father of our children. While it may never happen, I do not rule out the possibility of finding someone with whom I may want to form a relationship.'

'And how committed are you to make this happen?' I asked.

'One hundred per cent' was her prompt response, 'but as I mentioned earlier, I would want you to talk to David.'

'Would he be ready?' I checked.

'I will persuade him to come here and meet you,' she asserted.

And she succeeded in getting him to Singapore.

He was a man far removed from the person I had visualised him to be. He seemed much older than Emma had suggested to me. The wrinkles on his forehead seemed more pronounced due to his baldness.

'David, what do you want to say about this situation?' I asked him when we met for the first time.

'It's unfortunate that we are where we are,' he stated, 'but it could not have been any different.'

Emma was right. He did have a way with words.

'What options do you see in front of you?' I questioned.

'There is only one option possible, and that's also the only option that I would want to take,' he said emphatically.

'And that is?' I helped him continue.

'I love Emma dearly,' he confessed, 'and I love her even more now for the way she has handled the situation. I would never want to let go of her. I respect Laura as a friend and companion and don't want to see her hurt. I owe my life to my parents, for they have made me the person I am today. And of course, I adore my children and wouldn't even consider the possibility of being away from them.'

He looked at me and waited for my response.

'So, what would you want to happen?' I questioned.

'I would be happy if everything remains the way it was before my father revealed the truth to Emma,' he professed.

'And what if Emma doesn't want it that way?' I quizzed.

'I will keep trying, and am sure I will be able to convince her one day,' he asserted.

I continued with my line of questioning that day and for a couple more days before my last session, when I invited both of them for a joint session.

'One thing that comes out very clearly from my discussions with the two of you is that you love each other dearly,' I stated. 'David was the only person who knew what was happening, and the choice to continue was his. If the present situation could have been avoided, it would only be because of David. But he did not do that. Who am I to say whether that was right or wrong? However, one thing is clear. He made the decision with the purest of intentions. He has been true to your relationship and never made you feel deprived of his love and companionship. But does that absolve him from the blame? I don't know. What matters in the end is not what is right and wrong but what is acceptable to the two of you. There will be implications for every decision you make, but I am sure all of them can be addressed once you are thinking clearly, which is what I have been working on.'

Having listened intently, David and Emma spelt out their choices. Most of what they wanted matched, except for Emma wanting to end their relationship and thereby avoid any physical intimacy.

In spite of her magnanimity, one thing was certain. She felt a deep sense of hurt which would not go away easily.

'I respect your decision,' David said, 'but I will continue to woo you and win back your love for me.'

The two protagonists had made a decision. Whether it was right or wrong, only time would tell. But they were now ready to move on with their lives.

For the next few years, the routine continued. After every three months, David would spend a couple of weeks in Bali. He would live in a hotel and spend time with the children. He would have conversations with Emma. His attempts to woo her continued but were not yet successful. She went back to living her life, restoring the business and indulging in her children and the rest of her family. Twice a year, she would accompany the children to Switzerland, where she would live in Lucerne, and they would live with his parents. Laura accepted the children but never attempted to bond with them.

Through all this, Dewi grew very close to her mother, whereas Intan idolized his father. David paid special attention to their children's education. When Dewi finished her middle school, he took her to America and enrolled her in the Los Angeles high school.

On her first day in her new school, the professor called Dewi to the front of the class.

'Good morning, boys and girls,' she addressed the students. 'We have a new student joining us today. Please welcome Sofia Bussinger.'

Dewi smiled as her real name was called out.

# 14

One glimpse of her and I could tell that she was Emma's daughter. She had inherited her looks and the striking blue eyes from her mother.

'I am so glad that you agreed to see me, Dr Preeti,' she said with gratitude.

'It's you who has travelled a thousand miles to come here,' I responded with a smile. After her introductions, I asked her, 'Sofia, what brings you here?'

Sofia narrated the story of her life, ending with the suicide attempt.

I had a few sessions with her and helped Sofia understand her own self, her desires, and their drivers.

Sofia had been part of the events in her parents' life. While she was too young to understand what was happening, her mind was at an impressionable age, when beliefs and desires become ingrained. My sessions with her revealed that she was very close to her mother and she had seen her suffer. Subconsciously, she had made up her mind that it was her father who was the reason for her mother's condition. As she grew older, she realised that her mother desired physical intimacy, which she was denying herself due to her failed relationship. When Sofia was at an age where she was attracted to boys, this latent desire of physical intimacy of her mother came to the fore. She may not even be thinking with her own mind when she would get into these relationships, which probably explained the multiple pregnancies. Abortions take an emotional toll on any woman, and so it did with Sofia. For the last two years, she had been grappling with the unconscious desire for physical intimacy and the emotional turmoil which resulted from her actions.

My role was to bring this into her awareness and disconnect her subconscious desires with her present self. Sofia returned to Singapore a few more times, and my sessions helped her not only bury the past but also isolate its impact. She developed an increased sense of resilience, which was needed as she lost her job at the media house and was required to start her career all over again, in addition to putting the pieces of her personal life back together.

Today, she is associated with another prominent media company and is slowly making a mark there. She is not dating anyone but is more confident about what she is looking for in a relationship.

I was aghast when I finished this case.

Emma and David had made certain decisions some ten years ago, having considered all the implications that were obvious at that point in time. What they had never imagined was that the impact of the events from their life would cascade to the next generation.

Sofia was a girl in her preteens when her parents were going through a troubled period in their relationship. While Emma and David tried to insulate their children by not bringing up the subject in their presence, it had not helped. What became apparent from my sessions with Sofia was that the impressionable minds of children are affected not only by the behaviours and emotions of people around them but also by the energies and vibrations they exude.

I had administered therapy to the mother, and after many years, also to the daughter. What was intriguing was that the reason for their needing therapy were the same, although it had manifested itself in different forms. While I had worked with the mother and seemed to have helped her get over her troubles, I failed to realise at that time that its effect had already spread and planted weeds in the people around her. This case has only strengthened my belief in the laws of nature.

> *The Laws of Nature are just, but terrible. There is no weak mercy in them. Cause and consequence are inseparable and inevitable.*
> —American poet and educator Henry Wadsworth Longfellow

# CHAPTER 6

# THE MASTER

## 1

He was 11 years old.

He had accompanied his father, or rather, he was forced to accompany his father to this strange place.

After travelling many hours in a train and then a rickety hand-pulled rickshaw, he found himself in a room filled with fifty odd people, each of them in different stages of ecstasy. They were chanting, singing, and dancing all at the same time. His father made him sit in a corner and joined the frenzy. The dim lights in the rather congested room added to the mystical aura.

He would rather have been playing with his toys than travelling this long distance from their home on the outskirts of Wulai, a small village in Taiwan, to where they now were. The few minutes in the strange place only seemed to reinforce that feeling. Just when he was wondering what this fuss was all about, things began to happen.

'The Master is here,' someone shouted from the front, and everyone in the room cheered in unison, 'Hail the Master.'

Clad in a white robe which covered his generous frame from shoulder to toe, the Master had a presence. His greying hair which was tied in a ponytail, and his long beard gave him the appearance of the wizard from some comic book. The Master had striking eyes, which seemed to pierce through anything that he fixed his gaze on.

He came and sat on the raised platform at one end of the room. The room went silent. The Master opened his mouth and in a pleasant voice addressed the group of people gathered there. While the little boy did not make any sense of what was being spoken, he was mesmerised by the sound of his voice. It was so warm and alluring. It seemed to bring a sense of calm in his otherwise turbulent life.

That was his first encounter with the Master, and somehow the little boy knew that it would not be the last.

## 2

April is sakura (aka, cherry blossom) season in Singapore. The island is turned into a sea of pink as the trumpet trees bloom at this time of the year. Although the weather can get crazy with the heat of the morning punctuated by thunder showers towards the evening, I love this season. I increase the duration of my morning runs along the streets lined up with these colourful trees. Sipping a cup of tea while gazing at the lovely flowers from my bedroom window is something I indulge in very often during this period.

A cold shower after the morning run had refreshed me, and I was looking forward to the day ahead of me. Sandra was already at her desk as I entered the clinic.

'A lovely morning, Dr Pandit,' she greeted me with a beaming smile.

'A lovely morning indeed,' I responded warmly.

'Your first appointment is at 11 a.m.,' she reminded me.

'Thank you, Sandra,' I replied. 'And I suppose it's a new client, right?'

'Yes,' she answered referring her diary. 'It's a gentleman named Mr James Wong.'

I love the days when I have to meet a new client. Every person comes in with his own story, which is unique in its own way. Understanding human behaviour has been my passion, and every human being is an amalgamation of a complex set of emotions which influences behaviours. The ability to see beyond the physical presence of the person is what has enabled me to help the many clients who come to me with their problems.

It was 11:10 a.m. when he walked in. He was wearing cream trousers and an oversized white shirt. His unkempt hair, ill-fitting glasses, and unpolished shoes suggested that he was not a person who seemed to care about his appearance. He was rather young, probably in his midtwenties.

'Hello, Dr Pandit,' he said softly. 'I am James Wong.'

I shook his rather limp but soft hand and greeted him, 'Good morning, Mr Wong,' and I enquired, 'Can I call you James?'

'Yes, of course you can,' he said without any hesitation.

'So, what brings you here, James?' I enquired.

His hands were tightly clasped and feeling each other, which is usually a sign of nervousness. Well, it is very rare that a confident person walks into my clinic for his first session.

He finally spoke.

'Dr Pandit,' he said haltingly, 'I am seeing a psychiatrist, Dr Lee Chi Kin. He referred me to you.'

'Oh, is it?' I remarked. 'I am acquainted with Dr Kin.'

I had met Dr Kin at one of the conferences on mental health, and we had shared a dislike for artificial medication as the only cure for mental illness.

'What was the reason for your visits to Dr Kin?' I asked.

He continued haltingly, 'Things are not too well in my life. I am jobless and very low on confidence. I feel very lonely and miserable. I have been sick most of the time. My GP said that I am suffering from depression and suggested that I see a psychiatrist.'

'How long have you been seeing Dr Kin?' I asked.

'It's been two months now, and nothing seems to have changed,' he said despairingly. 'I am confused and unable to think logically. I feel like hiding from crowded places. I get self-conscious and always get the feeling that people are observing me. I am afraid people will notice that something is wrong with me. I am afraid that people will think that I am less confident.'

'And what makes you think that?' I enquired.

'Because my eyes look unusual. My dressing and hair are not good,' he said with a sigh.

I had observed that one of his eyes was slightly smaller than the other, but it was nothing so glaring as to be a cause for self-confidence issues.

'Please continue,' I prodded him.

'All the stress made me start drinking. I have been drinking quite a bit. When I was working, I was not able to perform. I always had the fear that I will not be able to do my tasks. I could not develop the courage to ask for help, fearing that others would ridicule me for not knowing my job. I would take a lot of breaks and drink to take my mind away from work and …'

'And what, James?' I asked softly.

'I have been running away from reality,' he said after a pause, and I could see tears welling in his eyes.

'What do you mean?' I questioned him in a bid to make him talk more.

'I want to run away from all this. But don't know where to. I cannot face myself. I have started drinking and smoking every day. I buy skincare products to make me look better and maybe to make up for what I lack. But Dr Kin tells me that this is not an external thing. I may be inadequate inside. I am constantly flooded with negative thoughts, fears which turn into anxiety. I am more anxious when I have no activity. Even when I was working, I would feel that I was not good as my colleagues at managing the team. I do not want to look uncomfortable in front of my boss.'

James went on with his tirade for the next quarter of an hour, and I did not hear anything positive about himself in that time. Clearly, he was suffering from a severe loss of self-esteem.

I did not want to stress him beyond a point in the first session. I wanted first to make him feel comfortable about sharing his personal details with me. I made a note of his medications and made a mental note to speak to Dr Kin to get a medical perspective to the case.

I suggested some breathing exercises which would help him stay calm before we decided to meet the same day in the following week.

### 3

It was almost a year before the little boy could visit the place again.

He was looking forward to seeing the Master again. The place was bigger than what he remembered from the last trip.

There were more people, and the atmosphere was even much more charged up.

After a long wait of more than an hour, the Master appeared. His appearance was the same, but this time, he was escorted into the room by two young boys, who were wearing similar robes but blue in colour. Chants of 'Hail the Master' echoed throughout the room. The intoxicating smell of incense filled the place apart from the smoke, creating an unintended haze.

When the Master spoke, everyone listened. His voice was as mesmerising as he had remembered from the last time. After speaking for a few minutes, he beckoned to a person from the crowd and asked him to come onto the platform. The whispers in the crowd suggested that we were about to witness something magical.

The Master made the person sit beside him in the lotus position and signalled him to shut his eyes. The Master did the same. Silence ensued. The little boy was surrounded by people much taller than himself, and he had to keep shuffling his position to catch a glimpse of the two figures through whatever gap he could find between the people in front of him.

For the little boy, the next few minutes were nothing short of a miracle.

The two men started levitating from the ground. He watched with bated breath and eyes wide open. The spectacle lasted for a few minutes before they slowly descended back to the ground accompanied by the collective gasps of every person who had the good fortune to be there.

The Master opened his eyes and made some gestures. The other man opened his eyes and looked around, seemingly unaware of what had transpired some moments ago. He bowed his head to the Master and strolled back into the crowd.

The crowd chanted, 'Hail the Master.' The little boy joined them. He had never seen anything like this before in his still young life of 12 years.

## 4

James was in a dishevelled state when he walked in for the next session. He gave the appearance of someone who had not slept for many days.

He sat on the chair, and his gaze was moving all around the room. His hands were pressed hard against each other as he leaned forward with the elbows on his thighs.

'It's a pleasant day, isn't it?' I stated with a broad smile.

It was almost like lightning cutting through his clouded mind and seemed to catch him by surprise.

'Ah!' he gasped and continued seemingly without a clue to what he was responding to.

I gave him time.

'Can you please put on that light?' he said suddenly, pointing to the white light on the ceiling.

The lamp next to my table is normally lit during my therapy sessions since it creates the right ambience. This was an unexpected request, and I fulfilled it. The enhanced lighting in the room seemed to fill him with some energy, and he sat upright on the chair.

'Did you sleep well last night?' I asked him.

'No,' he murmured. 'I couldn't sleep. I ... I ... was scared.'

'Of what?' I queried.

'I ... I ... don't know,' he muttered.

'Were you alone?' I enquired.

'Yes,' he quipped.

'Was it related to something that happened during the day?' I asked.

He continued, seemingly ignoring my question.

'I was scared,' he said, again reflecting on the previous night. 'He will come and take me away.'

'And he is ...' I helped him continue.

He remained silent.

On a whim, I switched off the ceiling light and asked him, 'Do you see him now?'

He covered his face with his hands and gave out a scream. 'Please put the lights—'

'Do you see him now?' I asked.

'Yes ... please save me,' he pleaded.

It was time to lead him to the therapy chair.

For the next thirty minutes, James dug deep into his past and in fits and starts shared his story.

'When I was about four or five years old, my parents would leave me with a babysitter. She would put me to sleep and then watch movies in the living room. One night, I couldn't sleep, so I stepped out of the bedroom and peeked into the living room. There was a movie playing on the television. I watched from behind the curtains. Suddenly with a loud bang, he appeared. He had long hair, which was curled towards the end. The skin of his face was peeling off. His eyes were big, and his teeth were stained. I watched from behind the curtains. He roamed the streets at night and sneaked into houses of children who were bad. He killed them and drank their blood. I let out a scream. My babysitter scolded me for being a bad boy. I ran back into my bedroom. I couldn't sleep that night and many nights thereafter. One night, as I was climbing up the staircase to our apartment, I saw him. He had a big knife with blood dripping from it. I let out a cry and ran to the apartment. I kept banging the door until my mother opened it. I put my head in her apron and did not want to let go of her lest the knife man get me. After a few nights, when I had to get my bicycle from the basement, I saw him again. I was terrified. I saw him again in the carpark of my apartment. Every night when I sleep, I have nightmares where the knifeman is roaming the streets searching for me.'

He started shaking. His body started trembling as if he was witnessing the nightmare.

'No, no, no,' he screamed. 'He is out to get me.'

I just let him be and slowly brought him back to the present.

He was scared of the dark. Many children personify darkness by giving it a shape and identity. This is a very common phobia among children but generally eases off as the person gets into his teens. Clearly, that was not the case with James.

There also may have been a correlation between his lack of confidence and this phobia.

'What's your normal day like?' I asked as a diversion and also to help me plan the activities that I would want to engage him with.

'I don't have much to do.' He sighed. 'I have to attend interviews on some days and that is it.'

'What about friends, your close family?' I asked, adding loneliness to the list of his challenges.

'Catherine was my best friend, and she disappointed me,' he said in anger.

'What did she do?' I asked.

'She called me a lunatic,' he yelled, 'as if I have lost my mind. She is much older than me, and I looked up to her as an older sister. When she said that, even Bobby and Jerry laughed at me. They mocked me. I don't want to see them again—ever. How could they do that?'

His body started trembling again but this time in anger. He was someone who had little control over his emotions.

'Do you have a girlfriend?' I asked.

'No' was his monosyllabic response to even the friendliest question.

'What about your close family?' I probed.

'No, I don't have anyone,' he screamed, and this time it was loud.

I waited for him to calm down. I needed to engage him in some activity which would keep him occupied as well as provide him with an opportunity to enhance his self-esteem.

'Do you swim?' I asked James after he had a glass of water and seemed more at ease.

'I can't swim,' he replied.

'Let me reframe that,' I suggested. 'You don't know how to swim now but could swim if someone taught you how. Am I right?'

'Yes,' he said with a faint smile.

'James,' I explained, 'just by changing the way we look at things and the words we speak, we can make things different.' I added, 'And It can even bring a smile to someone's face.'

James nodded his agreement.

'Would you know of any swimming clubs near your residence?' I enquired.

'I remember seeing a board of a Swimming school,' he recollected.

'Your homework for this week is to visit the school, get yourself enrolled for some swim lessons and get started,' I instructed him.

He did not seem convinced.

'Why do I need to learn swimming?' he questioned.

I looked him in the eye and said sternly, 'James, you have come to me to escape from a situation that you find yourself in. You need to trust me and my methods. They may seem unusual, but my experience suggests that they are effective.'

He stared at the floor, probably considering my instruction. 'OK, Dr Pandit,' he finally said, 'I will do it.'

His voice was nothing more than a murmur, but I could sense some conviction in it.

It was time to end the session.

## 5

The little boy's next visit was after eight months.

With every visit, the place seemed bigger and the crowds larger. There was more music light effects, and drama as the Master made his appearance in his trademark white robe. Nothing about his appearance, however, had changed over these two years. The two boys in blue trailed him and stood behind him in reverence.

After his customary address, a person on the microphone screamed some instructions in Chinese. From what the little boy could understand, the person was urging someone with a problem to come on stage. There was some jostling in the crowd, and a few men clambered up onto the platform as the Master's bodyguards kept the crowd at bay. The person with the mike urged each person to spell out their problems. Over the din, the little boy could only hear that one of them had a limp and another person was born deaf.

The Master raised his hand and beckoned the crowd to be silent. The men, who had climbed up the platform, were standing behind him. After a few minutes of meditation, the Master rose and walked to the first person and touched his forehead for a moment. He repeated this action with all the others. He took his position back on the platform and went back into meditation. With a sudden flurry, he lifted both his hands and pointed them to the sky, and there was a puff of smoke which engulfed the platform. Once the smoke cleared, there was a frenzy. All the men on the platform were screaming what seemed like shrieks of joy. They were all shouting, and the little boy could not make any sense of what was happening. The frenzy lasted for some time before the person with the mike came back on the platform. He requested the crowd to be silent as he spoke to one of the men standing. The man was panting, and in between his heavy breathing, he screamed, 'It's a miracle. My limp is gone.' He walked around the platform with pride and joy as he showed off his newly acquired attribute. Every person on the platform seemed to have experienced a similar miracle.

'Hail the Master!' the person with the mike hollered, and the crowd responded. There was an orgy of noise for the next hour.

Just like the last couple of times, the little boy's father asked him to wait in a corner as he joined the queue of people who went up the platform for a tryst with the Master. He watched with awe as the Master sat regally on his throne and went about his business. The little boy was desperate for an audience himself, but he did not have the courage to ask his father.

On the journey back home, however, he decided that he would somehow convince his father to let him fulfil his now obsessive dream of meeting the Master.

## 6

I have always believed that the environment influences a person's behaviour. I had met James within the confines of my clinic until now, and my intuition suggested that a change in setting might help bring a different facet of his life to the foreground.

Sandra called James during the week and informed him that the next session would be held at a different venue. The setting would be the coffee shop of the swimming school immediately after his swimming session on Tuesday of the following week.

I reached the place a good thirty minutes early. The advisor guided me to the training pool, where an instructor was helping eight adults fall in love with water. One of them was James. More than developing an affinity to water, this was my attempt to help him fall in love with himself.

I watched from a distance as James went through the paces. I would need to give him a few more days before this activity would start having the desired effect on him.

'How are you enjoying the swimming lessons?' I asked when we were seated at the coffee shop.

It may have been a delusion, but James seemed more alert than the other times I had seen him, when morose would have been a more apt description.

'It's fine,' he replied without any noticeable sign of excitement.

It was going to take time.

I had deliberately chosen a corner of the coffee shop which was silent, and the place was only occupied by a couple of other people anyway, which was an ideal setting for me.

I jumped straight to the point. 'James, tell me about your childhood.'

'I have lived all my life in Singapore. My father was a worker at an electronics company, and my mother was a teacher. They are retired now and live in Jakarta. I went to a public school and then attended junior college, but I dropped out without completing my graduation.'

'And why was that?' I asked.

'I was never interested in studies,' he reminisced and after some thought added, 'And the environment at home did not help either.'

'Please go on,' I urged.

'I had the worst father that anyone could have,' he blurted. 'He took away my childhood. He would hit me and fight with everyone around him. I never had a family.'

He was finding it difficult to speak as he recollected his bitter past.

I tried giving him a different perspective. 'Every father loves his children. Maybe he never showed it.'

His temper rose.

'Do you show your love for your child by throwing away the birthday gift he brought for you?'

'Why did he do that?' I asked.

'You need to ask him,' he screamed 'I was only eight years old. Imagine what I would have felt at that time. He never bought anything for me. He did not save any money for his family. No one in our family liked us because of him.'

The tears started flowing.

'He had a terrible childhood as well,' he stated suddenly. 'His family was very poor, and he grew up in very difficult conditions. That experience has made him a bitter person.'

That made sense. People who go through a difficult childhood either take it up as a challenge and ensure that their children don't have to live a similar life or succumb to the circumstances and let it affect the rest of their life and those of their family.

'Do you think I could study in such a house?' he yelled.

I waited for a few minutes and then continued, 'What about your mother?'

'She did not protect me from my father. She never stopped him from hitting me. I was all alone.'

'Why did she not stop your father?' I asked.

'I guess she was weak,' he said in anger. 'He would hit her as well. But she had to at least stand up for me.'

He shared more instances of his parents' behaviour which seemed to have affected his childhood. The clarity with which he narrated those incidents gave me an indication of how deeply ingrained they were in his psyche. From what he had shared, James seemed to have had a difficult childhood, and up until now, he had let that affect him adversely. In most cases, however, the individual paints such a grim picture based on his own perspective because that is the only lens through which he has seen the world. I now had to help him step back and see things differently, as well as not let the memories of these incidents affect his present and future.

I ordered coffee for the two of us and allowed him to have a few sips of the refreshing beverage before making my point.

'I have another suggestion for you,' I stated.

'Let me tell you a fact,' he said, seemingly ignoring my statement. 'I have never been as physically exhausted as I have been in these past few days. I am required to take a nap during the day.'

'That's good,' I responded and added with a smile. 'Let's hope it also drives the big monster away at night.'

It was a rarity, but James gave the hint of a smile.

'Have you heard of Vipassana?' I asked.

He gave a blank look.

'It's a form of meditation,' I explained. 'It is supposed to have a positive impact on our minds and bodies. I practise Vipassana meditation myself and have benefitted from it.'

He nodded.

'I strongly recommend you start practicing this form of meditation,' I stated.

He was listening.

'I will give you the address of the Vipassana International Centre,' I continued. 'Do visit them and enrol for their ten-day meditation course.'

He nodded.

I believed that the swimming and Vipassana meditation would slowly help James improve his self-esteem. I was also hoping that the meditation would wean him off from the excessive drinking that he was indulging in. However, I still needed to get to the bottom of his sleepless nights and help him get rid of the dark memories.

Were there more of these memories? I needed to find out.

## 7

The little boy, now a teenager, finally mustered courage to confront his father and state his intent to meet the Master. It turned out to be easier than he had expected.

'Maybe the Master will be able to drive some sense in you' was his father's response.

He did not mind the cynicism. His mind was already racing ahead to the time when he would come face to face with the Master.

This time, the teenager did not mind the arduous travel, the heat and the hunger. He did not even pay any heed to the even more extravagant paraphernalia that preceded the entry of the Master.

He was finally the second in the queue and after what seemed an eternity, he had his audience with the Master.

'And we have a smart young man here,' stated the Master when the teenager came face to face with him.

'He was very keen on meeting you,' the teenager's father said. 'I did try to tell him that the Master does not give an audience to children.

'He is not a child anymore,' said the Master with a faint grin.

'Yes, Master,' said his father, relief writ large on his face.

'What do you have in mind?' the Master asked him.

'I want to become like you,' the teenager said even surprising himself with that display of confidence.

His father was aghast and pinched his arm.

He grimaced in pain but stood his ground.

'You definitely can,' said the Master and the grin became wider. 'Are you ready to do what is needed?'

'Yes,' he shrieked in anticipation.

'I want you to let him get what he wants,' said the Master to his father.

'What do you mean?' asked his father, unsure of where this was leading.

'Leave him with me,' the Master stated nonchalantly.

'What?' His father gawked in disbelief. 'How ... is it possible?'

'It's definitely possible,' said the Master, 'once you consider it as a possibility. Your son will stay here for a year and learn the secrets of life. I have a dozen young boys like him who are my students.'

For the teenager, the last few minutes were magical. He had come there in the hope of spending a few minutes with the Master and ended up with the opportunity to learn from the great man for a year.

His father, on the other hand, was still trying to figure out what had just transpired. The man had been referred to the Master by a friend almost five years earlier when his life was in doldrums. He had been visiting the Master for the last four years but had not really seen the effect of the magic, as so many others had. He had been getting his son along since he hoped the Master would make a boy out of him. However, when the moment came, he was too ashamed to speak out. He had made up his mind that this would be his last visit to the Master and hence had relented to his son's request. Thereafter, everything happened so fast that he was left wondering what he could have done.

With the decision made, the teenager was led to his humble abode, which he would be sharing with three other boys. He was given two sets of clothes, very similar to what he had seen on the boys who accompanied the Master earlier.

He was on top of the world and strongly believed that his life was about to change.

It was definitely about to change, but not in the way he would have hoped.

# 8

When he walked in, I observed that James' gait was as feminine as I had seen him the first time. His gestures and hand movements also hinted at this tendency.

After the initial pleasantries, I asked him, 'How are your swimming lessons coming along?'

He couldn't resist a smile as he declared, 'I can swim now.'

'That's good. I am talking to a swimmer now,' I quipped.

'Did you enquire about the Vipassana course?' I asked.

'Yes, I did,' he replied. 'They have a ten-day course starting in a couple of weeks. I have enrolled for that course.'

I could see the first signs of self-confidence from the way he was experiencing a sense of pride and joy even in these small achievements.

'James, we have met a few times now,' I said when he was on the therapy chair. 'You have spoken about your parents, but

I have not heard you talk a lot about your friends. You did talk about Catherine, Bob and Jerry. Tell me more about them.'

He reacted instantly. 'They are not my friends anymore.'

'Who are your friends?'

'I don't have any,' he stated bluntly.

'Tell me about your relationships,' I persisted.

He was silent. 'I don't want to talk about them,' he blurted.

'And why would that be?' I asked.

He did not answer.

'James,' I said, 'I want you to go back to the moment you walked in here for the first time. Why did you come here?'

'I know,' he murmured. 'I should never have come here.'

'That is not going to give you a better life James,' I stated sternly. 'There is a part of you which is frustrated with the life you are living, and it wants to break free. That part of you has seen enough of grief in your childhood and wants to see better days. It is that part of you which forced you to come here. It is that part of you which is forcing you to the swimming pool when you would rather be in bed doing nothing. However, that part of you is still weak and gets overpowered by the other part of you which does not want to change. This other part is so used to the horrible childhood, the binge drinking and chain smoking that it is constantly rearing its ugly head and making you waste your life even more. James, life is all about choices. You have been making the wrong choices so far. This is a chance for you to finally start making the right choices. Don't hold back now.'

That tirade hit the bullseye.

His emotions burst out in a flood, and he was completely out of control.

'I do want a better life … I do want a better life,' he muttered repeatedly in between his wails.

'Nothing is lost, James,' I explained, 'but you need that small part of you to become bigger and be ready to face whatever the other negative part may throw up in front of you through old memories, heartbreaks, and broken relationships.'

He acknowledged my statement with a nod of his head, but the tears kept coming.

I allowed him to let out his grief.

'Tell me about your relationships,' I urged when he seemed to have regained control.

'I never had a relationship until I was twenty,' he declared. 'In college, everyone I knew was in a relationship. The peer pressure led me to ask her out for a date. I was surprised that she agreed.'

'Who was she?' I interrupted.

'Alicia,' he replied. 'She was in my class. Not very beautiful but intelligent.'

'And?' I helped him to continue.

'We went out for some time, but nothing happened,' he stated.

'Meaning?' I asked.

'I realised that I was not sexually attracted to her,' he said haltingly.

'Please continue,' I urged.

He continued, 'When I was twenty-two, I realised ...'

He stopped.

'James,' I prodded, 'what did you realise?'

'That I was attracted to boys,' he screamed.

It was as if a volcano, which had been simmering all this while, finally erupted.

'I got into a relationship with Lim,' he stated. 'He was my boyfriend for almost two years. We were buddies and spent a lot of time together. But I was not happy. I got bored and left him.'

I remained silent, waiting for him to continue.

'I got into a relationship with a guy who was twenty years older than me,' he continued, 'but he had lied to me about his age, and I left him when I found out about it. I spent time with a few more guys, but it did not last beyond a few weeks. I was never happy.'

Here was another reason for his poor self-esteem. He was attracted to men, but he was ashamed to admit it, not only to the world but even to himself. He was in a denial mode. By not accepting his sexuality, he was constantly in a state of unrest. The other thing that intrigued me was that all his relationships were short-lived. There was something else, apart from his denial, which was not allowing him to continue with any relationship.

It would require another session for the secret to be revealed.

## 9

The teenager had been living in the small tenement with his three roommates for a couple of weeks now. During this period, he had to follow a strict regime—waking up at a specified hour, cooking his own meals, spending time with a tutor who taught some religious principles, running errands for the Master and his staff before retiring for the night. In these two weeks, he had not even seen the Master let alone learning by him.

Was this the magical life that he had dreamed about?

That night, just when he was about to get into bed, there was a knock on the door. The teenager opened the door to find Chia-hao, one of the Master's staff members there.

He asked the teenager to come with him.

They walked in the darkness until they came to the Master's abode. This was a plush two-storied mansion with a huge iron gate guarded by a pair of security guards. Chia-hao spoke to one of the security guards and he let them in. A staff member opened the door to the mansion.

The teenager was confused and equally scared, wondering what was happening.

Once inside, the teenager was spellbound with the grandiose on display. Chia-hao asked the teenager to wait there and went away. The other staffer asked the teenager to follow him as he walked up the stairway. He reached a door on the upper floor and slowly opened it. He asked the teenager to enter while he himself left the room and closed the door.

The teenager was alone in the big room. He looked around. In the dim light, he could see a bed in the centre of the room, while a shelf and a cupboard lined up the two walls.

The teenager was petrified. He was about to turn back and run out of the room when the door opened, and he could see the silhouette of huge person. As the person came towards him slowly, he realised it was the Master.

Instinctively, he bowed down and remained in that position. The Master stepped forward, gently put his arms around the teenager's shoulder, and said softly, 'You want to become like me.'

The teenager was dumbstruck. It slowly dawned upon him that he was standing next to Master. In the dim light, the Master looked menacing with his broad frame, white robe, long hair, and beard.

'I will give you all my magical powers,' he said gently. 'These powers are stored in every part of my body, and it will take a lot of time before they can get transferred to you. We will start tonight and do this many more times before you get all the powers. It is only after that you can start using them.'

The teenager could not believe his ears but everything about that setting was making him nervous.

The Master gently ran his fingers through the teenager's hair and slowly caressed his face.

The Master continued softly, 'You may feel something strange at first. That is because these magical powers are very strong. If you resist these feelings, then the powers will never come to you, but if you welcome them, you will get all the powers sooner than you expect. Are you ready for it?'

The teenager was trembling now but a part of him nodded.

The Master took the teenager's hand and started walking towards the bed. He sat on it and made the teenager stand in front of him. Slowly, the Master moved his hand over the teenager's face and down his body and started lifting the teenager's robes.

The teenager became stiff and moved back.

The Master held him more tightly and said, 'The powers will only get transferred when our bare bodies touch each other. Let these clothes not come in the way.'

He couldn't move and was trembling all over.

The Master held the teenager's hand tightly and with the other, he lifted the teenager's robes over his head. Without loosening his grip, he removed his own robe and threw it aside to reveal his naked body.

The teenager was horrified. He was old enough to sense what was happening here but was too weak to resist. He wanted to scream but could not find his voice. He wanted to run but his feet had turned to jelly, and the Master's grip was too strong anyway.

'You are a good boy,' the Master whispered. 'I will give you all my magical powers.'

The Master caressed every part of the teenager's body. The teenager was feeling a variety of sensations, but he had no will to resist. The Master continued whispering as he slowly but forcefully pulled the boy down on him. The teenager just let him have his way.

An hour later, the staffer took the wailing teenager back to his room. Along the way, he was warned not to speak to anyone about whatever happened that night, or else he would be killed.

Once the teenager was in his room, he shut himself in the toilet and cried the whole night. He was in a lot of physical pain, but the humiliation and shame were even greater. He confined himself to his room the next day. When his tired body drifted into slumber, he could see the silhouette of the Master in the dark room coming towards him and he would wake up with a scream.

It was after a few nights that Chia-hao turned up at his door again. This time, the teenager resisted but he was easily overpowered by the burly staffer and literally dragged to the mansion.

Despite his timid resistance, the Master bestowed his magical powers on the teenager again that night and for many more nights thereafter.

The teenager had nowhere to go. He had no money and the place was unfamiliar. He did not have the courage to do something different to escape the ordeal that he was facing every other night. He had come there to transform his life. His life had indeed undergone a huge transformation which he would not have imagined even in his wildest dreams.

It was only after a few months that the teenager could escape from the hell he was living in when his father came back to take him home. The Master's staff had threatened him many times during the past few months, and he was anyway too traumatized to share his ordeal with anyone.

During these months, the teenager had been at the receiving end of every kind of sexual act that could be imagined. The initial feelings of fear had shifted to shame and humiliation, which finally led to a morbid acceptance of everything that had transpired as a conspiracy of fate. Life made no sense to the teenager anymore. He completely disowned himself and his identity.

For the teenager, James was dead.

## 10

It took several therapies before the secret from his past came out into the open. I had to help him delve into his unconscious mind several times before he could piece together the events from those dark moments and narrate every gruesome detail of his molestation by the Master.

It took me awhile to gather myself when James had finished. The man had actually lived through a nightmare which he was terrified to recollect even in his thoughts. While the memories of those nights were confined to some dark corners of his mind, the associated feelings and emotions were manifesting in different ways. I could now explain his lack of self-esteem. He was too scared to even bring the image of the Master in his conscious memory, but his fears had created a fictitious monster and assigned the reason for his behaviour to it. It was ironical that the painful memories were so deep-rooted, yet his mind had confined them to some dark corner lest they come up as a conscious recall. Even if he wanted to, he could not have recollected those memories on his own. It required many sessions of therapy to bring them back into his conscious memory.

I made him say the words 'I was molested' many times to let him register that fact. Acceptance is the first step to any kind of change and the change that James had come to me for could not have been possible without these gruesome facts coming to the fore and him acknowledging them.

I could now work on reducing the impact of these painful memories on his current and future life.

For the next few sessions, I helped him detach himself from the events. Yes, he was molested, but there was nothing he could have done to prevent it once he had made the choice to live with him. I had to rid him off his shame and guilt. I had to restore his identify, which was so much more than what was taken away from him by the cruel man.

The swimming sessions helped in making him more resilient. I set targets for him to achieve in terms of speed and distance every week, and this helped create a sense of achievement. He slowly started gaining control over his life. The Vipassana course helped him understand himself better. In the session after the course, he revealed that he was more aware of his sexuality now and ready to accept himself the way he was.

It was after many more sessions spread over the course of the year that James walked into my clinic with a beaming smile.

'Dr Pandit,' he exclaimed, 'I have found the perfect job. I feel so confident about myself and my abilities now. That helped me crack the interview.'

'That's wonderful, James,' I said with a smile. 'Good luck to you.'

At 26 years of age, he still had his whole life ahead of him.

# CHAPTER 7

# THE FORGOTTEN YEARS

## 1

The sound of a gunshot pierced the silence that had shrouded the place.

The eight boys dived into the pool a few milliseconds apart from each other. Considering the competition on show, this could mean the difference between a podium finish and the also-rans (or, in this case, the also-swams).

This was the final of the 50 metres freestyle race for under 13s at the National Schools Swimming Championship.

The boy in lane 3 had taken an early lead, but the boy in lane 4 and the favourite in Lane 5 were just an arm's length behind. The rest of the field were being left behind. The boy in lane 3 reached the 25-metre mark first, but his rather feeble push at the turning point resulted in the favourite taking the lead.

The crowd cheers loudly as all the boys stretch their every muscle, and in less than a minute, they reach the finish line just a few milliseconds apart from each other. The announcer screams into the microphone to make himself audible. The winner of the 50-metre freestyle in the under-15 category is Joshua in lane 5. The crowd applaud generously. Their favourite had won. A close second in lane 4 is Li Wei. And the bronze medal goes to Ashraf Ali in lane 7. All the boys come forward to congratulate the podium finishers, except the boy who swam in lane 3.

Adrian was sulking in a corner with his face between folded knees.

'I knew it,' he was berating himself. 'I am not good enough. I deserve this.'

## 2

Back home, Adrian skipped lunch and shut himself in the bedroom of the house where he lived with his parents and a younger brother, Luke. He kept playing back the race in his head and cried himself to sleep.

The loud banging of the bedroom door woke him up. He jumped out of bed, ran to the door, and opened it.

'What the fuck are you doing in here with the door locked?' his father growled as he marched into the room. The smell of alcohol followed him.

'Dad!' Adrian gasped, trying to find the right words. 'I ... I was sleeping.'

'You lazy son of a bitch,' his father snarled. 'This is not your private room for you to be having a siesta in broad daylight. Did you win today?'

'Dad ...' he murmured. 'I was leading ... but ...'

'But what?' His father sneered 'You lost ... again.'

Adrian remained silent.

'You good-for-nothing jerk,' he shouted, pointing his finger at Adrian. 'Have you ever won anything in your life? You are coming with me to the pool again from tomorrow, and this time, I don't want to hear any excuses.'

Adrian dreaded the thought of being in the pool with his father. Every time it had happened in the past, the session in the pool had been a disaster for him. His father would make him swim until he couldn't move any more. It always ended with his father cursing him for not being good enough and screaming at him in the presence of others. Adrian knew his limitations and did not want any reinforcement of his shortcomings.

'You will not get any dinner today,' his father bellowed. 'That's what losers deserve.'

'Daddy!' Adrian pleaded. 'I am hungry. I ... I ... did not have my lunch. Please ... please ... I am hungry.'

That seemed to irk his father even more. He pulled out his belt and, without any warning, let it rip.

As Adrian lay in bed that night, he was feeling a plethora of emotions. He was feeling the pain of the belt's hard leather on his back. He was feeling ashamed for not being good enough at anything. He was extremely angry with his father, whom he did not just hate but despise. He was frustrated since he did not see any escape from this hell. He was too weak to take any drastic actions anyway.

Strangely, Adrian also had a sense that he deserved this punishment by his father. Why, he was not sure.

Adrian cursed himself and his destiny as he rolled in bed with hunger pangs. He only had his pet cat, Kitty, and of course, his nightmares for company. As long as he could remember, Adrian had been having these nightmares, and it occurred again that night.

***

He is naked and running for his life on the streets trying to escape a huge crowd which is trying to get hold of him. The crowd seems very angry as they shout expletives at him. His legs are aching. He is running out of breath, but he cannot stop. Some people from the crowd close in on him. As he looks over his shoulder, he can see his father, his mother, and his Uncle Joseph in the crowd, and they look angry—very angry. He is exhausted and cannot run any further ... Everything is becoming a blur ... He cannot see clearly ... He is losing consciousness. He can hear the heavy breathing of the people in the crowd ... And then everyone in the crowd extends their arms long and grab him. They begin to strangulate him. He is not able to breathe ... He is gasping for breath ... And then he wakes up.

***

He begins to sweat profusely; his breathing is heavy, and his head is reeling. He quickly runs to the living room to check if the door of their house is locked. Breathing a sigh of relief that the angry crowd will not find him here, he sits down on the couch in the living room. It takes a while for him to realise that he was seeing a nightmare. He dreads going back to his room lest the nightmare returns to haunt him.

# 3

Theirs was a modest household. Adrian's father, Kurt, was a janitor in one of the many offices that had Orchard Street in their address. His life was a sad story, having been born in a poor family, missing out on a proper education, and seeing his dream of becoming a football player never getting fulfilled. He married

Kim at a very early age in the hope of finding a companion for life. Alas! Kim had her own history of misfortunes, which had gotten the better of her, leaving her fighting many battles with her own mind. With his personal and professional life in doldrums, Kurt turned to alcohol for comfort at a very young age. In his intoxicated state, he would let go of his frustrations on anyone who happened to come in his way.

When he had two sons, he hoped that they would live his dream of becoming a sportsman. From a very early age, he pushed them into various sports and demanded excellence at every step. His older son, Adrian, liked the action but lacked a killer instinct. His younger son, Luke, hated sports, and his poor physical health did not permit him to indulge in physical activities anyway. They would never be able to fulfil his dreams, which was a grouse he would always harbour.

Kim had a history of her own. She lost her father at an early age, and when she was in her early teens, her mother was identified with cancer. While insurance took care of her treatment, all the other household expenses fell on her head. She had to drop out of school and work to support their family, which included her two younger sisters. She saw her mother suffer a lot as the dreaded disease sucked out every ounce of her energy. Her mother passing away was a relief more than grief.

Like every girl, she hoped to marry the proverbial prince who would help her build the life of her dreams. Kurt seemed to be that person. She fell for his strong physique and handsome looks, and it was not too long before she married him. Kurt had dreams of becoming a professional football player, but it soon became an obsession. He did not seem to understand that he lacked the skills to succeed at the highest level. His lack of focus led to him getting fired from multiple jobs, and very soon, he started taking out his frustrations on his wife. He would hit her if she did not let him have his way in bed. He would not allow her to work in the fear that she would earn more than him. If a sober Kurt was maniacal, a drunk Kurt was a terror.

The daily torture at home began having its effect on Kim and she suffered a nervous breakdown just a few years after Luke was born. Even after some medical treatment, she continued to be hysterical and would lose control of herself from time to time. To make ends meet, she had enrolled herself with one of the employment agencies who offered her odd jobs from time to time. On these days, the boys would go to their aunt's house after school.

Today was one of those days.

Adrian had received the grades for one of his class assignments that day, and it was an F. He dreaded the thought of facing his father. As he stepped out of school, he asked Luke to proceed to their aunt's house citing some work. The very thought of going home made him nervous. With a blank mind, he started wandering the streets without any idea of where he was going. He kept walking for more than a couple of hours, and it was only when hunger got to him that he realised he was lost. Not knowing what to do, he started shivering and fainted. Some passers-by called the ambulance, and he was rushed to the hospital. The doctors administered some drugs to improve his blood pressure, and an ambulance dropped him at his aunt's place. His aunt was livid with him for his indiscretion. When their dad came to pick them up and heard about the incident, all hell broke loose.

'You stupid son of a bitch,' he shouted at Adrian while holding his arm tightly. 'So you are thinking of running away, are you?'

'Ah …' he screamed in pain. 'I am sorry, Dad … I did … didn't know … what I was doing.'

His aunt intervened, 'Kurt, it's OK. He has learnt his lesson. I am sure he will not repeat this.'

'You bet he won't,' Kurt said, seething in anger. 'I will make sure he remembers this day.'

In a flash, he removed his belt and started hitting Adrian mercilessly. The pleas and attempts of the family fall on deaf ears. After a few minutes of his ruthless show of anger, Kurt finally stopped and threw the belt away.

Adrian remained crouched in the corner and wept uncontrollably. His entire body was shaking with fear and pain. His aunt comforted him, and when he was stable, he gave him some food to eat.

That night, he kept wondering ...

'What have I done to deserve this hell?'

'How can someone be so ruthless and cruel?'

'I will run away from here ... but where will I go? ... I know Uncle Joseph lives on the other side of town, but I am sure he will inform my dad ...'

He kept tossing in bed as his mind is contemplating all the possibilities. Suddenly, a thought arose: *Maybe I deserve this life ...*

This thought is like a beam of light piercing through a cloud of smoke. *I may have done some bad things and ... and ... probably this is a punishment.*

*But ... but what have I done? Was getting an F in my exam so bad?*

Nothing seemed to make sense to his young and inexperienced mind until another thought arose: *What if I end all this?*

Just the thought sent a chill through his spine. *Yes ... I will end all this. I will ... I will jump in the sea and kill myself. Yes, this life sucks.*

By the time he cried himself to sleep, Adrian had made up ·
his mind. He had to wait for an opportune moment.

# 4

That opportune moment came in a couple of weeks.

The school had arranged a study tour to the Jurang Bird
park. As the guide was explaining the characteristics of the rare
Shoebill birds, Adrian's thoughts were elsewhere. When the
group dispersed for a short break, Adrian slipped away from the
group and made his way to the exit. He checked his pockets to
feel the few dollars he had managed to find in his mother's purse
that morning. Mustering some courage, he even walked up to
the service desk at the park's entrance and asked for directions
to the beach.

As instructed, he boarded the Line 98 bus, and in a couple
of hours, he found himself at the East Coast Park.

He started walking towards the water, but a sense of
nervousness started creeping in. As he neared the sandy part of
the beach and the vastness of the ocean came in full view, the
enormity of what he was trying to do suddenly dawned upon
him. He was scared—really scared. His hands and feet started
turning numb. As he kept staring at the vast ocean, he felt as if
the waves were coming closer towards him and about to drag
him into the water. It suddenly seemed like the crowd of people
from his dreams who were out to get him. They were coming
closer and closer and about to engulf him.

With a shriek, he suddenly turned around and started
running, fear written all over his face. He kept running blindly
for a long time, and just like the previous day, realised he was
lost. Even in that state of panic, he had the presence of mind to
approach a policeman and ask for help.

As the police car was taking him back to school, he was hoping that the school authorities would not have noticed his absence, but he was wrong.

As the police lead him to the principal's office, Adrian's heart skipped a beat as he saw his parents waiting outside. His grade teacher was also there with them. He felt weak in his knees, and the shivering returned. He stopped and tried to turn around and run, but the policeman was holding him tightly. His face was a mask of fear as he saw the angry face of his father. For a moment, he cursed himself for not having ended his own life. It would not have been worse than what he imagined would follow.

The principal issued a warning and let him go.

As they walked out of the school, his father held him by the neck but did not say a word. They hailed a cab and reached home. As soon as they entered, his father rushed to the kitchen and returned with a chopping knife. He held the knife close to Adrian's neck, brought his face very close to Adrian's, and whispered menacingly, 'I have had enough of you and your games. Let me end it right here. Shall I?'

His breath was in Adrian's face and the tip of the knife pressing into his neck. In spite of all the torture he had endured so far, Adrian had never felt as much fear as he felt at that moment. He did not even realise that his trousers were wet.

While his regular trysts with his father continued, the relationship with his mother never left the ground. She would be in her own world, rarely in a state of mind to be her children's mother. Adrian was so involved in his own woes that it never dawned upon him that his mother was going through traumatic times of her own, until that day when he came face to face with a new reality.

The day, in fact, started off rather well. Skating was another activity which Adrian indulged in regularly. That day was the selection trials for the university skating team, and Adrian had just performed a brilliant routine to get into the top three, which was necessary for the qualification. The remaining two skaters needed an exceptional round for them to get through. As each of them finished their routine, Adrian waited with bated breath for the scores to be announced. And when that happened, he was over the moon. He jumped up in joy and hugged his mates. At that moment, he was so happy that all his personal troubles seemed irrelevant.

An elated Adrian reached home to see everyone in a state of panic.

'What happened?' Adrian asked searchingly.

A panting Luke held him close 'Brother! Mummy took an overdose of sleeping pills … Something has happened to her,' and he pointed to the bedroom.

'What?' Adrian gasped 'What … how … what are you saying, Luke?'

His dad was on the phone, possibly calling an ambulance. He rushed to the bedroom, and there she was on the bed, lying motionless. Adrian bent down and touched her swollen face. He could feel that she was breathing but was not conscious.

He looked at their maid who seemed to be in a state of shock and asked, 'What happened, Nui Nui?'

'Madam took a lot of sleeping pills,' she replied. 'I found her lying on the floor and called sir.'

Adrian stared at the figure lying on the bed. Her face seemed so calm, without the stress lines that had become a distinct feature on her forehead. As he kept watching, he realised that this was probably the longest time he had seen his mother from such close quarters. He kept wondering, *Why did she take this extreme step?*

And then a thought came like a bolt from the blue: *Oh my God! I am the reason for this. I was so happy this morning. I am not supposed to be happy. Did my mother receive this punishment because I was happy? I don't deserve to be happy.*

He took her hands in his own and started wailing. He continued to cry as the ambulance arrived and shifted her to the hospital.

Adrian's mother survived, but the incident left a deep scar in his mind, which would continue to haunt him for many years. Adrian's teenage years passed him by in the midst of an overbearing and disciplinarian father, a mentally sick mother, a physically weak brother, and a head full of guilt, doubts, fears, and suspicions. He did manage to complete his graduation, but the travails of his growing years had a significant impact on his personality. He was completely devoid of any self-confidence and would even fear making eye contact with people. His body would start to shiver at even the slightest provocation. He would be suspicious of everyone and everything and never grew to trust anyone, including his own self.

He was good at swimming and skating but never quite made the cut from being an amateur to developing into a professional sportsman. The constant pressure from his father did not help either, and he developed a hatred for these and any other sport.

His personality and lack of any social connections did not help him make friends, and of course, there were no girlfriends. He had this ingrained belief that he was responsible for everything that was happening in his life, and he had no right to be happy. After his graduation, he failed in multiple interviews, until he found himself serving tea in a café. But even this tenure was short-lived, as his nervous demeanour led to him spill tea on a client. He got fired.

Adrian had fallen in a deep hole, which had probably been dug by others but was being made deeper by him.

It was this Adrian who walked into my clinic that day.

As he recounted his past over multiple sessions, I could read his body language like a book. Every trait of his was manifesting itself without any attempt on his part to downplay them. During the conversations, he would constantly look around as if to ensure that no one was overhearing him. His entire body would tremble as he narrated his experiences. One thing that struck me was that he would blame himself for almost all the situations that he would find himself in. It was as if he had this deep sense of guilt, and that all that was happening was a form of punishment which he had to endure.

There was something that he had done for which he had a lot of regret, but the problem was that even he did not seem to know what it was. Likely, the answer to his present situation would need me to unravel this mystery. But I sensed that it would take time.

During our initial sessions, I kept peeling one layer at a time, slowly making him feel comfortable with me and with himself. I helped him recount all that he wanted to share and comforted him to a point where he would want to continue talking. I encouraged him to socialise and urged him to engage in physical activities like swimming and running, which he seemed to like. I wanted him to look at the future with hope and expectations rather than dwell on the past with trepidation and fear.

In one of the sessions, I gave him the opportunity to dream about the future. I gave him a writing pad and asked him to write down his aspirations. I was not surprised to see him struggle. He had this deep-set fear that wishing for something good meant inviting more troubles. I even gave him suggestions to develop a more confident body language. All these interventions did have a positive impact but only slight. I still needed to peel off many more layers to reach the real Adrian.

## 5

Psychotherapy is a means of helping a person dig deep into his or her memory bank and trace the origins of current behaviour patterns. In many cases, the person is displaying a certain behaviour but there is nothing in his conscious memory to justify that behaviour. In such cases, I resort to intense therapy where I help the person to delve deep into the subconscious and find relevance. If done in the right manner, and with the support of the person involved, many facts do come out which can be stitched together to draw inferences.

When Adrian came to the clinic that day, I felt that today was the day. He seemed calmer, and the frown on his face was missing.

'Hello, Adrian,' I greeted him. 'You look good today.'

A smile appeared.

'Thank you,' he responded. 'I went for a swim today.'

'That's wonderful Adrian!' I exclaimed. 'How are you feeling?'

'You were right—it felt good,' he admitted.

'Adrian,' I said, 'I want to set you free from the invisible shackles that are binding you. But it can only be done if you want to do it. Are you ready?'

The smile disappeared.

'What are you going to do?' he asked, scepticism writ large on his face.

'Nothing we have not done before,' I assured him, 'but with a little more intensity. I want you to put your mind to it. That's all.'

'O-O-OK,' he responded, still seemingly apprehensive.

I asked him to lie down on the couch and over the next few minutes guided him to a state from where he could access his subconscious mind while constantly observing his breathing and body language.

'Adrian, I want you to pose a question to your subconscious mind through the power of your thoughts,' I said softly when I sensed he was ready. 'Ask, "What am I sorry about?" Bring this question in your thought and seek the help of your being with a deep sense of gratitude.'

He remained motionless.

'As your subconscious mind starts giving you the answers, tell me what you see, what you hear, what you feel. The answer may not seem obvious, but there will definitely be an answer.'

I waited as his breathing ebbed and flowed and slowly fell into a pattern.

'What can you tell me Adrian?' I asked.

'I am in a car with my father and my cousins. My father is driving too fast. I am telling him to slow down, but he ignores me. I am scared … my cousins are scared. I am feeling embarrassed that my cousins have to experience this.'

He was on the right track.

'I feel contempt towards my dad,' he remarked.

'Why contempt?' I asked softly.

'Because he always gets away with his other self—the unruly, forsaken attitude. He has no regrets. How can he do that?'

I urged him to continue. It was like sifting through many folders on a computer until I find the folder that had the answer. The problem was that I was not sure what I was looking for.

'What do you regret, Adrian?' I continued. 'Bring this question in your thoughts.'

Many moments of silence ensued. I had to be patient.

'What are you sorry about, Adrian?' I asked again.

'My dad is driving. I am with this girl I like. She is scared. I did not like his driving, and I approach him about this a few days later. "You are putting our lives at risk," I tell him. He seemed to acknowledge it, but with his continued silence. However, after a few days, he does the same thing after his drinks. I am really upset. I feel sorry for my friend and decide never to go with my dad in his car again.'

He shares a few more instances about his father, which seemed very trivial. He could recount a few instances with his mother. None of them seemed to have been the reason for his regret.

'My mum is using sarcasm to mock my brother and me for our habits. She is mocking us now. She is calling me a hypocrite for going to church and serving God but not obeying her or pleasing her expectations. She is so contemptuous and condescending.'

Many more sessions continued in the same vein. I engaged him in multiple activities in an attempt to give him a sense of accomplishment, which in turn would increase his self-worth. But nothing seemed to be working. Adrian would pursue an activity for some days and then get bored with it.

It was more than three months since we began our sessions; in most cases, there would be a shift visible by this time. Not with Adrian. Every bitter memory of his was either about his father or mother.

I had to use a different approach. I opened the writing pad on the desk and opened the page on which Adrian had written what he most wanted to do.

There, written in capital letters was the word 'Sorry.'

I kept staring at the word. What started as an open and shut case seemed far more intriguing. He seemed to have recounted all his bitter memories. What was he sorry about?

And it struck me. Why was I harping on the bitter memories? What if the regret is due to a happy memory? The more I thought about it, the more I sensed it could be a possibility. In the three months we had been talking, he had hardly ever mentioned a happy memory. His teenage years and beyond were difficult by his own admission. What about his early childhood?

The train of thought led to a plan for the next session.

## 6

He was on the couch again. So vulnerable, so fragile.

'Adrian,' I said softly when he was ready for the therapy. 'I want you to bring into your thoughts the happy memories from your childhood. Go back to the moments when you were really happy.'

His breathing suggested that his thoughts were going somewhere. He would have to sift through the many layers of pain before he would find the happier memories he was looking for. I had to ensure that he remained committed to the task. I kept talking to him, encouraging him and urging him to do the same to his subconscious mind, which had the missing pieces to the puzzle.

Thirty minutes went by, and nothing happened. I remained patient and continued to probe. It was close to the hour into the session that the moment arrived. His words came out in fits and starts.

'I am cutting my birthday cake. Everyone is singing for me. I am excited with all the gifts I am getting …

'I open all the gifts. Wow! This gun is so big … I thank my uncle for it …

'I am running all over the house and shooting everyone. This is so much fun.

I could see from his expressions that he was in a happy place, which is exactly where I wanted him. I had to determine his age to connect the pieces together.

'How old are you today, Adrian?' I whispered in his ear at an opportune moment.

'Aunt Maria, I am 4 years old,' he screamed.

He continued speaking with a pause after almost every word.

'I am in the bedroom, and I am unable to sleep …

'I want to play with my toys, but my father will be angry …

'I look around, and Nicole is lying next to me. She is sleeping. She … she is so tiny. I … I … I touch her face …

'Her skin is so soft …

'I take her small fingers in my hand and feel the tenderness of her palms …

'I take her hand and rub my face with it. It feels so nice … I keep doing it …

'I move my hands from her face and over her body to her feet … They … they are so tender. No wonder Nicole cannot even walk properly …'

He smiles.

'I keep stroking the soft legs gently, and it feels so nice.'

Where was this leading to? Who was Nicole? His body language suggested that he was enjoying the moment that his subconscious mind had brought to the fore.

He continued with his voice becoming huskier, 'When I was at Uncle Joseph's place the other day, I had entered the bathroom …

'The maid was bathing Nicole ...

'I stood there and watched ...

'I noticed something different about her ... I became very curious.'

The session was heading in a direction which I had never imagined.

'I am now excited that I could now see it again ...

'I ... I slowly lift her tiny skirt ...

'Oh, no! She ... she is wearing diapers.

'*What do I do now?* I wonder, and then I move my hands over them and find the prickly thing which is holding it together. With some force, I slowly pull the prickly thing and the diaper is free ...

'Why is she different? Why ... why does she not have what I have? Does it grow after some years? After all, Nicole is only a year old.'

*Oh! My dear Lord*, I thought. Nicole was just 1 year old! And Adrian himself was only 4? *This cannot happen.*

It was my turn to feel a chill running through my body. I was feeling sick, wondering where this was heading, but I had to stay put since this was probably the answer to all my questions about Adrian.

'I ... I slowly touch her ...

'She is soft all over ...

'I sit up and pull down my pants ... I want to see what is so different ...

'I touch my thing and then ... I touch hers ...

'It feels so strange, but it also feels nice ...

'*What if I touch her thing with mine?* I wonder ...

'I slowly move towards her and rest my legs on hers ...

'Gently, I use my hand to guide my thing so that it caresses her thing ...'

I can see the pleasure in his face. He seemed to be experiencing a sense of joy which had never surfaced during the last three months.

'I am feeling a tingling sensation all over my body ... and ... and I am liking it.

'I keep doing it for some time, and strange things are happening to me. And then ...'

*Haven't I heard enough?* I thought. This was one of the most bizarre things I had ever heard in my long career. *How could this ever happen?*

His expressions suddenly changed to one of anxiety. His voice comes out in gasps. 'Shit! I hear the front door opening ... I can hear Papa's voice ... Oh, no! Will he scold me? I quickly stop what I am doing and sit up. I somehow cover the diapers and pull down her skirt. I jump onto my side of the bed and close my eyes just as the bedroom lights come on ...

'I am breathing heavily ... I am afraid they will know I have done something ... I close my eyes more tightly ...

'I can hear Mama and Papa arguing about something. After some time, they switch off the lights and get into bed ...

'Thank God ... I can now go back to the moment ... I don't know why, but I feel so happy. I want to do it again, but I somehow feel that I should not do it when my parents are around.'

He stopped speaking, but his expressions suggested he was still in the ecstasy of the moment.

*Does he even realise the enormity of what he had just shared?* I thought. *Why did this incident never come up in our earlier discussions? How can an incident like this be forgotten?* Well, Adrian may not have recollected the incident, but the impact of the incident on his psyche remained. I didn't want to, but

I had to listen to what transpired next. I still had to find out: Who is Nicole?

Intuitively, I took out my voice recorder and began recording what Adrian was about to say. I might need to replay it for him, since he was not likely to remember most of what he had said so far.

After a few moments of eerie silence, Adrian started speaking again.

'I have been waiting for this moment for many days now, and ... and ... finally, I have it ...

'My parents are away ... and Uncle Joseph is in the other room watching TV ...

'Nicole is playing with her Barbie doll ...

'I go near her and ... and rub my hands gently over her face ...

'She is smiling ...

'I lead her to a corner of the room ... I make her sit.

'I slowly pull her pants down ...

'She is giggling ...

'I ... I undo her diapers ...

'There it is again ...

'I ... I slowly touch her thing ... and I feel the tingling sensation again ... and ... she continues to giggle ...'

He smiles.

'Probably, she ... she is feeling the same tingling sensation that I am feeling now ...

'I keep caressing her thing and ...

'I feel happy that she is also enjoying it ...

'*How do I touch her thing with my thing?* I wonder ...

'I slowly push her upper body ... forcing her to lie down on her back ...

'I rest my legs on her thighs and … and … I turn my body
…'

'My thing is now near hers … and I bring them together …'

I was horrified. Probably even that adjective seems simplistic
to convey my true state of mind at this moment. I did not even
want to hear this any further. *How can a toddler …?*

With a start, his voice again becomes louder, and his body
language suggests a state of panic.

'Oh no! I can hear footsteps outside the door. It is probably
my uncle … I quickly pull my pants up and then I tidy her up
… She is giggling all the time …'

'But … but I feel my uncle will scold me if he sees us like
this … The door opens.

'"What are you naughty children doing?" My uncle is
smiling as he comes into the room.

'I am breathing heavily … I am scared that he will punish
me …'

He comes near Nicole and picks her up in his arms. "Why
is my little baby giggling?" he asks her in a childish tone.

'I say to myself, *I know why … but this will remain our little
secret …*

'"And what have you done to your diapers, you naughty
girl?" he playfully chides her …'

The next quarter of an hour was the most difficult for
me. I could not bear to listen. I was now disgusted. But I did
not have a choice. The answers to everything that Adrian was
experiencing in his adult life seemed to lie in his narration.

Adrian narrated a few more similar incidents, which
suggested that this horrific game had been played over a long
period. I was relieved when I felt that I had heard enough, and
it was time to bring him back to the present.

I was speechless, with a number of emotions running through my head, but Adrian seemed oblivious to all that he had spoken. When he left, I went through my notes and felt even sicker. I was happy that I had a recording.

I helped myself to a nice cup of tea and sat back on my chair.

*Does he not remember anything about these horrific events in his life?* I wondered.

Selective memory is a person's ability to remember certain information and not remember other information. This type of memory implies a certain amount of intentionality behind it. It's a choice our brain makes, based on the emotions associated with events. Someone who experienced abuse when they were young might not remember what happened in full detail. The brain helps them to forget traumatic moments that would bring tremendous pain. Selective memory is like a protective layer created by the brain to control the flood of emotions.

However, it has been well documented that the avoidance of certain memories or experiences can leave complicated emotions that have nowhere to go. Just because the event has been forgotten does not necessarily mean there will not be ramifications. Most of the strong emotions experienced during the event remain. And without any associated event to fall back on, the emotions may lead to incoherent behaviours.

Was this a case of selective memory?

I rolled back the clock and started visualising my interaction with Adrian since the first time he came to me.

He was nervous, always wary of who may be listening. He was always concerned about the door being closed. His recollections were all about the bitter experiences of his teenage years. All along, he would keep making self-deprecating remarks. And importantly, the one thing he wanted to do was say sorry. To whom, he was not sure.

There is a possibility that the horrific events that he had recounted would be fresh in his memory during his growing years. After all, they were happy memories for him. At some stage in life, he would have been educated on the human body and the concept of sex. He would then have realised the seriousness of the playful act and may have been shattered. He would have felt a lot of shame and regret. A sense of fear about being found out would also have creeped in. He was by nature a very timid person, and hence the option of being open about it to his family never arose.

Like it happens with many others, he would have convinced himself that the events did not happen. Repeatedly doing that over some time led to the condition of selective memory, where the event was erased from the conscious memory but the strong emotions of pain and regret remained. There is a possibility that Adrian felt a sense of shame without knowing why. He would have felt a deep sense of regret without knowing the reason. He would have felt the urge to apologise without knowing to whom. He believed that he deserved punishment for what he had done and that everything happening in his life was part of that punishment. This also explained the nightmares that Adrian would have frequently. He was always living in the fear that the whole world was going to find out about his misdeeds and punish him even more.

Things seemed to be falling into place now. What remained was to bring this into Adrian's awareness and start his rehabilitation.

## 7

When he walked in, he was no different from all the sessions that we'd had over the past so many months. There was no indication that the therapy of the previous week had any impact on him. He seemed oblivious to the storm he had created in my therapy room.

'Adrian,' I asked, 'how are you feeling?'

'Fine, Dr Pandit,' he responded softly.

'We had a very intense therapy session last week,' I said. 'Do you remember any of the things that you shared with me?'

He thought about it and replied, 'I vaguely remember it was something about my childhood. I don't remember clearly … but I did feel very light that evening …'

I leaned forward and addressed him, 'Adrian, you came to me with a problem. You were not doing well in your job. You felt you were not good at anything—almost worthless. You shared all the events of your difficult growing up years, your troubled relationship with your family. You have not shared anything about your early childhood. Do you remember any events when you were four or five years old?'

His fingers started playing with each other, suggesting anxiety.

'That's a long time back …' he said as his gaze shifted to the ceiling. 'I don't really remember anything clearly …'

His anxiety was growing, so I intervened.

'Our brain captures everything that we have been through from the first breath we take. Some of these memories remain in our consciousness and we can recount them whenever we need to. However, we lose access to these memories-either because they were very uneventful and hence did not warrant any association or because they may be traumatic, and hence, the brain pushes them into some deep corner so that the negative emotions do not affect our future lives. In some cases, we try and convince our brain that an event did not happen, and over time, the brain erases the event from our conscious memory.

However, all the minute details of our lives are etched in our subconscious memories, and they cannot be deleted.'

Adrian was listening intently.

I continued slowly to help him comprehend what I was saying. 'During therapy last week, I was helping you to search these dark corners of your mind and retrieve the memories which may no longer be in your consciousness. I wanted to know all the experiences from your past which may have led to your present situation.

'Are you with me?' I asked.

'Yes, Dr Pandit,' he replied. 'I can understand what you are saying.'

I sat back on my chair and asked him, 'Adrian, who is Nicole?'

'Eh!' he responded blankly. 'Nicole?'

'Someone from your family perhaps ...?' I helped him connect some dots.

'Oh, yes!' he exclaimed. 'Nicole is my cousin.'

That was like a stone being thrown in the midst of a flock of pigeons. All of them suddenly panic and frantically take off with a flutter of wings.

*Adrian was assaulting his baby cousin?* I gasped, as the very thought of it seemed repulsive.

Coming back to the moment, I asked, 'Where is she now?'

His response was immediate. 'She is studying in America.'

'And how is she doing?' I probed further.

'Why are you asking about Nicole?' He seemed confused.

'I will tell you everything,' I assured him. 'But first, answer me.'

He did not seem convinced, but he replied, 'She is a star. She is good at so many things. She is an athlete and has won many medals. She is a fabulous dancer and also good in academics. She has gone to America on a scholarship.'

He was obviously proud of his cousin.

'She is so much unlike me.' He smiled sarcastically.

'Adrian,' I leaned forward again, 'listen to me carefully. During therapy, you were recounting some events from your past. Since there was a possibility that you may not remember them, I took the liberty of recording what you were saying.'

He immediately got jittery and exclaimed, 'You said … nothing will go out of this room … Why have you recorded—?'

I quickly interrupted his outburst, 'Don't worry. I will erase the recording in your presence once we have listened to it. Is that OK?' I asked.

'Umm.' He nodded unconvincingly.

I removed the recorder and placed it in between us and pressed the play button.

What followed for the next thirty minutes was a display of an emotional roller-coaster. It was as if he were listening to a horror story, but in this case, he was the antagonist. He stared in disbelief at the recorder as he heard his own voice describing every detail of the reprehensible act.

By the time the playback was over, Adrian was a mess. He was on the floor, sobbing uncontrollably. He was muttering expletives to himself, and I could sense an outpouring of rage as he clenched his fist hard and banged the floor.

After all, this was an outpouring of more a decade of emotions which were seeking redemption. I was sure that this moment of truth would be his gateway to a new life.

It was now time for the corrective therapy sessions to begin.

Over the next few weeks, I made him realise that the events of his childhood were an inadvertent result of a child's curiosity. At that age, all children are curious about things around them.

In his case, he happened to be enamoured about something for which he was not ready and which had a bigger implication that was not obvious at their tender age. However, to Adrian's credit, even at that tender age, he seemed to have a sense that what he was doing was not correct and he needed to do it when no one was around. I explained to him that his suspicious nature may have been developed during that period. When he became more aware of the implications, he developed a deep sense of regret which exists to this day. The only issue is the reason for the regret was not apparent, since he had forced the memories of those dark events into some deep corner.

He could now speak to Nicole and reveal the details of her past, but was it necessary? Nicole was just a year old at that time and would not have any memory of those events. Also, in her case, this would just be another uneventful game that might not have merited a place in her consciousness.

Why try and plaster a wound which did not seem to exist? I encouraged him to go to church and confess with all sincerity. I asked him to express his deep regret in front of the Lord and absolve himself of any blame. I engaged him in activities like swimming. I encouraged him to accompany me on my weekend runs along the beach. I urged him to become more social, go clubbing on weekends, meet people and develop friendships. I also gave his reference to a few HR consultants and connected him with consultants who would help him improve his overall personality.

The process was slow, but after a year from the day that he first came to meet me, Adrian had undergone a transformation.

When he walked into my clinic that day, he was so different from the Adrian I had met a year ago. He was well dressed in a formal suit. His hair was trimmed and combed well into place. His walk was more assured, and his handshake conveyed confidence. He had secured a job a couple of months earlier, and he seemed to be happy with his work.

'Good morning, Dr Pandit,' he greeted me. 'How are you today?'

'I am well and so happy to see you,' I said with a warm smile.

'I have a girlfriend,' he said with a smile. 'I thought you should be the first person to know about it.'

'That's wonderful!' I shared his joy and enquired, 'How is work?'

'I am enjoying my work,' he replied. 'The people are good and helping me get acquainted with the company processes. I realise now that a positive personality ensures that more people come forward to help.'

'That's a good observation,' I acknowledged, and we both had a laugh.

He looked at me, and his eyes conveyed a sense of gratitude.

'Dr Pandit, I cannot thank you enough. My life is so much better now only because of you. I am more confident about myself. I have better clarity on what I want to do in life. All this would not have been possible without your help. Thank you so much.'

I accepted his appreciation and added, 'I was doing what a therapist has to do. The only person who should be credited for this transformation is you. You have convinced yourself that this life is a gift, and you need to live it by being happy and spreading happiness around you. You need to congratulate yourself for that.'

As I walked home that evening, everything seemed so beautiful. It always did when I know that I have made a difference to another person's life.

# 8

This was a bizarre case. Adrian's life was affected deeply by some events of his childhood, of which he had no recollections. The supposed victim in this case, namely Nicole, was not affected in any way, since she was too young at that time. Rather, in this case, the alleged perpetrator of the crime became a victim.

A few questions come up. Is Adrian guilty of a crime, or is he the victim? Who should be blamed for the situation that Adrian found himself in his adult life?

The most obvious response would be the circumstances which led to the situation. But that would mean brushing the problem under the carpet.

What about Adrian himself? Of course, he would have to bear some part of the responsibility, however naive he would have been at that age. Also, for a major part of his life so far, he had let himself become the victim of his own mind.

What about his parents? They need to shoulder a large portion of the blame for being oblivious to the mental state of their son over more than fifteen years of his life. Did their overbearing nature lead Adrian to perform the heinous act? Did they leave any channel of communication open for their sons to share their concerns? While Adrian was ensuring that his family would not come to know of his act, isn't it the responsibility of the parents to be more aware of what is happening in their children's life? There would have been at least some indications. How could they be completely unaware?

What about Nicole's parents? While nothing much was spoken about them, there would be very little they could have done about it. Again, were there no indications over the period of one year which would have been considered as suspicious?

Well, Adrian found a lifeline at an appropriate time. I do hope the millions of people like Adrian find theirs.

# CHAPTER 8

# GENERATION DECISION

## 1

'*T*halaiva ... *thalaiva*' (Boss ... boss).

The loud chants pierced the silence of the night or rather the early morning.

For the uninitiated, it was like a pronouncement of the arrival of a divine force. In this part of India, where movie stars are accorded the status of demigods, this scene was an annual occurrence signifying the launch of a new movie with the *thalaiva*, or boss, in the main lead.

Among the frenzied gathering at this popular cinema house was Nandini.

Nandini was so much like the thousands of starry-eyed girls who lived and breathed movies. Her sartorial sense, her overall sense of style, and even her vocabulary were inspired by the characters from the silver screen, and her affluent family background only made it that much easier. Much like the others in the crowd gathered there, she could give her life for *thalaiva*.

At the crack of dawn, the dozen priests gathered there began the chanting of hymns as the larger than life cardboard cutout of their superstar was bathed in milk. The many litres of milk literally going down the drain did not in the least bother Nandini, as she watched in awe at the imposing figure in front of her. She waited with bated breath for the doors of the cinema house to open, when she would be transported into her *thalaiva's* world. At this time of the day when the rest of the country was just waking up, the hundreds gathered there jostled for positions as they entered the movie hall like a flock of migrating wildebeests.

What followed for the next three hours was a cacophony of sounds, some from the movie itself but even more from the audience. The superstar's grand entry was greeted with thunderous applause, and every dialogue of his was cheered. His mannerisms were accompanied by whistles, and every punchline was followed by peals of laughter. The movie showed the superstar as a bad guy who turns good due to the influence of a girl who falls in love with him.

During the next few days, Nandini would watch the movie many times, and her excitement would remain just the same as it was when she saw it for the first time. At 19 years of age, she was in her second year of graduation. Education was never her priority, and she would just secure the minimum marks needed to get into the next grade. After all, she was born into a business family which owned many restaurant chains in the southern part of the country. Theirs was a traditional family which believed in upholding the family name before everything else. The youngest child of three, Nandini was the darling of the family. Educating the girl child was never a priority for the family, and hence, her academic pursuits or lack thereof were never scorned. She lived a life of entitlement amid the many luxuries that surrounded her. She was an average looker, and her pampered existence showed in her body proportions.

Like many girls of her age, she would visualise herself in the role of the leading ladies who were in the enviable position of being the focus of her *thalaiva's* attentions.

## 2

The month of July and August is considered auspicious in this part of the world, and the main bazaars would be teaming with people shopping for fineries. This was also the time of the year when the premier college in this part of the country hosted the prestigious inter-collegiate festival, which was an eagerly awaited social event in every student's calendar.

Today was the last day of the three-day festival, and a popular rock band was on stage belting out popular numbers to the delight of the large crowd of students gathered on the lawns. Nandini and her group of friends were letting their hair down as they danced to the music being played. As the music reached a crescendo, most of the crowd were on a high from the spirits they had consumed or from the adrenaline which would have consumed their being.

In the heat of the moment, Nandini's flailing arms landed on the face of the boy next to her. As she turned to apologise, the strong smell of alcohol emanating from him made her cringe. She decided against the apology and turned back to continue with her dance moves. The snub, however, seemed to trigger a hornet's nest. The boy and his group of brawny mates turned their attention on Nandini.

'What he growled.

Noting the tone of his voice, Nandini thought it better to tender the apology after all, and she muttered an 'I am sorry' under her breath as she continued dancing.

'Hey guys, the queen is saying sorry,' the boy said sarcastically as the others moved closer and almost surrounded Nandini.

Nandini's group of friends sensed the intentions of this group and stepped forward in support.

'She is saying sorry, my friend,' Nandini's friend Uma intervened.

'And I am not in a mood to accept it,' the boy responded nonchalantly.

'So, what is she supposed to do?' Uma asked him, slightly irritated by the arrogant response.

'She hit me here,' he said pointing to his cheeks, 'and I want her lips to touch the same spot.'

'Have you gone out of your mind, you b$%#@*&,' Nandini screamed upon hearing the boy's indecent proposal.

Anger writ all over his face, the boy stepped even closer and pointed a finger at her as he spoke. 'Hey! Mind your words.'

'Hey, mister,' Nandini responded aggressively, 'point you fingers at someone else. You don't scare me.'

Before anyone could react, the boy held Nandini's face and planted a kiss on her cheek.

'Remember this moment,' he remarked in a husky voice. 'I get what I want whether you want to give it or not.'

The boy's group roared with laughter.

Any other girl would have been shocked and embarrassed, but not Nandini.

Mustering every ounce of her energy, she swung her hand and responded with the tightest of slaps. In spite of being very well built, the impact of the slap made him take a few backward steps. The slap made such a huge sound that that the other students near them, who seemed oblivious to the altercation until that point, stopped to look.

'You hmmm....' she retorted. 'Now, you remember this moment!'

The boy, obviously under the influence of alcohol, stepped forward and held her neck between his hands.

'I will kill you, furiously. ' he muttered.

By now, a large section of the crowd had turned their attention to these two groups, and a few people stepped forward to restrain the boy while a few others were trying to free her from his grasp. Nandini's group of girlfriends did not want to create a bigger scene and dragged an angry Nandini away. As they were being pulled away, Nandini and the boy's fiery eyes were fixed on each other as if conveying a message: 'This is not the end of it.'

## 3

For the next few days, his face was all Nandini could see everywhere. She would snap at people on the slightest pretext. She hardly had a morsel of food. Her mind was preoccupied with the thoughts of revenge. She was not going to let him get away easily.

It did not take long before their next encounter.

Nandini hated social gatherings with the family. She would be at the mercy of the family elders who would have only one question.

'My dear child, when are you getting married?'

She would wonder, *How can calling her a child and talking about her marriage happen in the same breath?*

She could not help joining her parents for the wedding reception of their distant relative. As her parents exchanged pleasantries with all and sundry, she preferred to find herself a quiet corner, away from the pesky glances of their acquaintances.

As the function proceeded, an announcer came on stage and welcomed the orchestra, which was supposed to entertain the guests. The music started, and a young lady sang a popular song. The announcer then came back on stage and stated excitedly, 'We now have a wonderful singer, Rajan. He will sing a romantic song from the latest *Thalaiva* movie.'

Nandini was all ears now. This song was one of her current favourites. As Rajan came up on stage and started singing the first notes, Nandini's expressions suddenly changed. She got up from her chair and started walking towards the stage, all the while keeping her eyes fixed on Rajan. The reaction of the guests suggested that he was singing very well, but Nandini was not listening. When she was close enough to see Rajan, she let out a gasp loud enough for people around her to turn around.

Rajan, the boy singing on stage, was the same person with whom she had the altercation the other day.

She had been so obsessed with the thought of revenge that her whole body seemed to tremble with rage upon seeing him there. However, his lovely voice and the lyrics of the popular song he was singing, calmed her down.

'How can someone with such a romantic voice be so obnoxious?' she wondered.

The song was greeted with a loud applause, which brought Nandini back to the present and her anger resurfaced.

As the next singer started her song, Nandini stormed into the room where the orchestra team were seated. Rajan was taking a breather and was startled to see her there.

She went straight up to him and said loudly, 'Mister, how dare you show your face at our wedding?'

The sudden intrusion surprised the other orchestra members, and they turned their attention on Nandini.

Rajan was still at a loss for words since he had never expected to bump into Nandini there. His mind was already occupied with the songs he would be singing and did not want a confrontation.

'Look, lady,' he said in a soft voice, which was very different from the brash tone that Nandini had heard the other day, 'let's take this up after the function.'

'And why would that be?' Nandini continued belligerently. 'Are you afraid that the public will see your real image?'

'I don't have anything to hide,' Rajan responded with more than a tinge of irritation. 'You are blowing things out of proportion. We had an argument the other day. It's done and dusted. Let's forget about it and move on.'

'Oh! Looks like you get slapped very regularly,' Nandini said mockingly. 'That did not mean anything to you.'

Rajan was getting angry now. *What can I do to silence this stupid girl?* he wondered.

Oblivious to the verbal banter in the adjacent room, the announcer had announced the next song. When the singer did not turn up, one of the team members walked into the room. Soon, the announcer, who was also the manager of the orchestra, made a hurried entrance into the room and proceeded to calm things down.

Nandini was not going to back off.

'The only condition that I will let this orchestra go on is if this person apologies for his behaviour with folded hands,' she declared.

The manager pleaded with Rajan to do her biding for the sake of the orchestra. Sensing the lack of support for him, Rajan did as he was told.

As Nandini walked away triumphantly, Rajan went back to his practice.

What was to follow would change their lives forever.

## 4

The bungalow was decorated with flowers and completely lit. It seemed as if the festival of lights had come early this year. The affluent family was celebrating the birthday of their favourite child.

The who's who of the business world were present at the party. Nandini was draped in a grand saree and the ornaments covering her body would have added a few kilos to her weight. The culinary spread on offer could have fed an entire village for a month.

As the party went on well into the evening, a couple of uniformed waiters brought the trolley with the huge birthday cake. Everyone gathered around the centre table in anticipation. As Nandini picked up the knife to cut the cake, a loud voice made her stop.

Someone was singing her favourite song from the *thalaiva* movie. However, the sound was not coming from the speakers at the party venue. Nandini knew this must have been a surprise planned by someone in the family or her friends. It was not a recorded voice. Whoever was singing the song, though, was doing a wonderful job. She wanted to see the person right away. The melodious sound was coming from outside the house. Leaving the cake behind, Nandini followed the sound and reached the gate. The people followed her.

Nandini was stunned by what she saw.

A huge banner was pinned to the wall in front of the gate. The banner had the words 'I am sorry' followed by 'Happy birthday, Nandini', and standing next to the banner, with a mike in his hand, was Rajan.

Nandini just stood there unsure of the emotions running in her head. Her friends were cheering and singing along with Rajan. Her conservative family, however, seemed embarrassed by this public display of emotions, especially since it was by a boy for a girl.

When the song ended, Rajan bowed down on his knees and brought his palms together. This was so much like the movies and an ardent movie buff like Nandini was floored. For a brief moment, their eyes met. He moved his lips and whispered, 'Sorry.' She smiled in response and murmured, 'Thank you.'

While they were not audible, the feelings seemed to reach the intended recipients.

On the behest of Nandini's father, the security guards went up to Rajan and requested him to leave. Nandini and the guests went back in the house. The party continued, but the birthday girl's heart was not there anymore.

The next day, Rajan turned up at Nandini's college. He walked up to her as she entered and smiled.

'Hi,' he said softly.

'Hi,' Nandini responded coyly, which was so much against her normal self.

'Can I have a word with you?' Rajan asked.

'Yes.' She thought for a moment and said, 'Let's sit in the canteen.'

She signalled her friends to proceed and led him to the college canteen.

They picked up their coffees from the self-service counter and sat at a table in the corner.

'I hope you have forgiven me,' Rajan enquired in his now-familiar husky voice.

'Forgive you for what?' Nandini asked.

'For being a jerk at the concert,' he replied with a chuckle.

She joined him and added, 'And what about my performance at the wedding?'

They had a laugh recollecting the venom they had spewed at each other, and while it was never explicitly spelt out, they seemed to have forgiven each other.

Rajan became a regular feature at Nandini's college. Upon his arrival, Nandini would leave her group and proceed with him to the canteen. They would talk for hours before leaving for their respective homes.

Rajan was the only son of an auto driver. While his childhood was spent in poverty, things were beginning to look up for the family. He was good in academics and secured admission in the government engineering college. Presently in his final year of Computer Engineering, his family was looking forward to the day when he would secure a good job. Rajan was very ambitious and had dreams of becoming an entrepreneur one day. He had a lot of business ideas which he would share with his friends. However, by the end of the conversation, he would realise that these ideas would remain a dream for lack of finances.

Nandini and Rajan's many rendezvous in the college canteen did not go unnoticed.

When Nandini came home from college one day, her father confronted her.

'What is this I am hearing?' he enquired in a rather serious tone.

Nandini looked at her father, and his stare suggested something was not right 'What are you talking about Appa?' she asked hesitantly.

'I hear that you are meeting this boy a lot,' he retorted.

Nandini was very afraid of her dad. In fact, he was the only person in the family that she feared. Her dad had a bad temper and was known to throw the verbal kitchen sink at anyone who defied him. While he had never raised his voice at her, she would generally try and avoid him. Theirs was a truly patriarchal setup, and her father was the boss of the house and even their extended family, which included his four siblings and their respective kin. His handlebar moustache added to his regal presence.

'Appa ...' she muttered feebly, 'nothing like that. I have a few friends who are boys, and our group sometimes sits in the canteen when there are no lectures.'

'Nandini,' he said gently, 'I trust you. I only want to tell you that I am proud of our family traditions and values. I have allowed you to study and have not put any restrictions on you. But when it comes to our traditions, I will not compromise.'

'Yes, Appa,' she mumbled even as her feet were getting cold.

When Rajan reached Nandini's college the next day, she was not waiting for him. His calls went unanswered. He could not get any information about Nandini from her friends. When this happened for a few days in a row, Rajan was concerned. He sought out Nandini's friend Uma and requested that she visit Nandini's home to check her whereabouts.

When Uma reached Nandini's house, she was there. After a brief chat with Nandini's parents, she joined Nandini in her room. She grew pensive when Uma raised the topic of Rajan and narrated the conversation with her father.

'I am scared, Uma,' she confessed.

'Nandu, I think you are thinking too far ahead,' Uma said, 'You have only met Rajan for a few days. Get to know him better. You have to be concerned about what your father said only when you guys get into a serious relationship. Have you guys spoken about all that?'

'No way,' Nandini quickly responded. 'I do like him but have not thought about anything serious yet.'

'Exactly,' Uma exclaimed. 'All parents are emotional and old-fashioned. Even if a boy and girl talk to each other, they start assuming many things.'

'You are right,' Nandini concurred, feeling relieved upon hearing Uma's words. 'Let me first get to know him better and then see what happens.'

After some thought, she told Uma, 'It may not be appropriate to meet him in the canteen. When you meet Rajan tomorrow, tell him that I will meet him at the Guindy National Park gate at around 4 p.m.'

Their meetings now shifted from the college canteen to different parks in the city. Just like in the movies, she was enjoying this secret courtship period with Rajan.

It would not be too long before things began to get serious.

## 5

The setting was romantic. They were sitting in a park with flowers around them, mountains in the background, a river gushing nearby and a gentle breeze ruffling their well-styled hair.

'Will you marry me?' he asked her.

'I thought you would never ask,' she said with a grin. 'Of course, I will marry you.'

They broke into a song.

Nandini and Rajan were watching a movie where the lead actor and actress were having this romantic conversation. As the movie played out in front of them, Nandini could picture herself falling in love with Rajan, marrying him against the wishes of her family but everyone finally reconciling to the situation and living happily ever after.

It had been more than two years since they had started seeing each other. Rajan was an engineer now and working in a global IT company. Nandini had just become a graduate and was wondering what to do with her life.

After that initial confrontation with her father, there were no further discussions on this subject at home. She assumed that it would be at least a couple of years before the subject of her marriage would come up. She was about to be surprised.

'What are you doing this Saturday?' Nandini's mother asked her one evening.

Nandini was busy watching a movie on television and nonchalantly responded, 'Nothing.'

'OK. Then be at home,' her mother declared 'We have some visitors ...'

'Umm' was Nandini's muted response and she became engrossed in the movie.

Saturday arrived. Nandini had set up a dinner date with Rajan and had nothing to do during the day.

After lunch, her mother took her aside and said, 'Nandini, I had told you about the guests who are coming today. I want you to get ready by 4 p.m. Wear that blue saree, and also put some flowers in your hair.'

'Amma!' Nandini replied with some irritation. 'What guests? And why should I get ready?'

'I told you about them the other day,' she retorted, 'but where do you have the time to listen to me.'

'OK, Amma,' Nandini conceded, not wanting to get into an emotional argument, 'I will get ready.'

Nandini did as instructed by her mother and made herself comfortable in the living room. Her mother came and sat next to her.

'My dear child,' she said, 'you look beautiful today. We are expecting Selvan uncle and his family. His son has just returned from US after completing his MBA. He will be taking over the family business and—'

'And what, Amma?' Nandini interrupted, worried about where her mother was leading.

'And … your father wants you to marry him,' she blurted out.

'What?' Nandini screamed and stood up in a hurry. 'What are you saying Amma? How can you decide something like this without even telling me?'

'Would we do something which is not good for you?' her mother asked.

'Amma, please don't get into this emotional blackmail,' Nandini countered. 'This is my life, and I have to decide—'

'And what is my little baby deciding?' her father, who had just walked into the room, interrupted.

'Appa!' she exclaimed and turned her attention to her father. 'This is not fair. How can you decide about my life without even consulting me?'

'Nandini,' her father responded calmly, 'I know what is best for you and the family. Sundar is a good boy and is also the only son of my friend Selvan. They have a huge business, and this alliance will be good for all of us.'

'But Appa …' Nandini tried to explain when the sound of the horn suggested that the guests had arrived.

Her parents left the conversation aside and proceeded to welcome the guests.

Nandini ran into her room on the upper floor and closed the door. She threw herself on the bed and started wailing. She was not able to think clearly. Multiple things were going on in her head.

*I would be called outside soon. What do I do?*

*What if they accept our proposal?*

*How do I bring up the subject of Rajan with my father?*

In that moment of madness, panic took over. Nandini picked up her purse and made her way to the lower floor, tiptoed to the kitchen, where their cook was arranging some sweets in a plate, made her way to the back door, which led into the garden, and exited the house. She hailed an autorickshaw and headed to Rajan's house.

'What are you doing here?' a surprised Rajan asked when he saw Nandini at his doorstep.

She was trembling with fear and nervousness. She tried to speak but was at a loss for words.

Rajan asked her to wait outside while he picked up the keys to his bike. He drove her to one of the parks that they frequented.

'What's the matter?' Rajan asked once they were seated in one of the lonely corners of the park.

'Rajan!' Nandini said. 'My parents want to get me married.'

'What?' Rajan exclaimed. 'What happened?'

She continued, 'A boy had come to see me today.'

'And?' Rajan was now impatient.

'And I ran away,' she declared. 'I did not meet him.'

'What?' Rajan reacted even more loudly.

'What else could I do?' Nandini too raised her voice, surprised at his reaction.

He said, 'You could have just met them. It's not that you would have been married today. By running away, you have only made matters worse.'

'It's easy for you to say that but I was in the situation,' she continued to justify her actions.

'Look here,' Rajan said, holding her hands, 'you have to go back immediately and apologise to your parents. Tell them you developed cold feet thinking about marriage. It was a silly mistake.'

'How can you say that?' she retorted. 'My father will kill me if I go back.'

'What do you mean?' he said. 'You have to go back. What else can you do?'

They fell silent, and it began to dawn upon Nandini that what Rajan was saying was true. She had indeed panicked in the heat of the moment, and running away was not the best option.

It was a big showdown at home that evening. Nandini fell at her father's feet the moment she entered her house.

'Sorry, Appa,' she cried. 'I developed cold feet. I am not ready for marriage, and when you suddenly invited a boy home, I did not know what to do … I am sorry.'

As expected, her father was furious. His steely gaze suggested the pent-up anger inside him. It was frightening. She hugged her mother tightly and cried. It took some time for the temper to die down, but Nandini had to pay for her indiscretion. She had to give a promise to be available when the family visited again, and she would not leave the house without permission.

The immediate problem had been resolved, but Nandini knew she did not have a lot of time on her hands.

Having sensed the situation, Rajan was already planning the next steps.

## 6

Nandini's moments were now restricted, and Uma was their only intermediary. Through her, Rajan realised that Nandini's parents had managed the situation rather well the other day. They had given the excuse of Nandini's periods as the reason why she could not come out to meet them. However, there was every possibility that their next visit was just around the corner.

Rajan had a plan in mind but he needed to meet Nandini to make it happen. The opportunity came when Nandini's parents had to leave for an outstation trip. They would be away for a day, which meant that Nandini would be alone with her grandparents. Under the cover of the blistering afternoon heat, when her grandparents were taking a siesta, as were the servants in the house, Rajan slipped in. In the confines of her room, he laid out the plans.

When Rajan had left, Nandini started putting the plan to action. That night, at an agreed time, she sneaked into her parents' room. She searched for the keys to the cupboard and found them under the mattress on the bed. In the cupboard, she found some jewellery which she put in a bag. As instructed by Rajan, she rummaged the cupboard to find some of her documents. She found a couple of passbooks and chequebooks in her name, which she picked up. There was some cash as well which she took. She had already packed her stuff in a suitcase. Nandini was certain that her father had instructed the security guard at the gate to not let her out in their absence, so she had thought of something. Early in the morning, Uma came home in an autorickshaw, and Nandini loaded her suitcase into it.

'We are donating some clothes to charity' she explained to their security guard.

When the vehicle was out of the gate, Nandini came running and told the guard, 'Brother, I forgot one small bag in the living room. Can you please go and get it?'

As the Guard went inside the house, Nandini stepped into the autorickshaw and they drove away.

While there was an element of fear, Nandini was also excited at the way things were unfolding. Much like in the movies, she was leaving the riches of her parents and going into the arms of the one she loved. Her parents would be angry and devastated, but she was sure that they would come around after some time. Doesn't that happen in all movies?

They drove straight to the marriage courts, where Rajan was waiting with one of his friends. At 11 a.m. on that fateful day, the district magistrate pronounced them husband and wife in the presence of their friends.

They proceeded to the police station and submitted the marriage certificate with a written application that they were getting married by mutual consent and their family should not make any attempt to find them.

They went to the railway station and boarded the train which took them to the hill-station of Ooty.

While Nandini's family was struggling to find legal options to annul this marriage, Nandini and Rajan consummated their love in the pleasant surroundings of the hill-station.

As the train chugged its way back to the city, Nandini gazed at the world outside. The last few days had been a blur. She was now stepping into this new life with Rajan. She knew that Rajan's family was poor and hence she would have to make some adjustments in her lifestyle. But that would be temporary. Rajan had promised her that he would be starting his own business very soon. Once that happened, money would pour in, and they would start living a lavish life. She believed him. After all, doesn't it happen so often in the movies?

She couldn't have been more wrong.

They reached the city and headed straight to Rajan's house. His mother asked them to wait at the door and brought the traditional *aarti* (a brass plate on which camphor is lit) to welcome them home.

Rajan took her inside his modest one-room house. The living room was cluttered with a lot of stuff, like old newspapers, a bottle of water, a towel just lying around. A bed with a slightly torn bedcover occupied most of the space available and doubled up as a sofa. A steel cupboard next to it and a table made up the furniture in the room. A small television set was hung on the wall. The adjacent kitchen seemed big enough to accommodate only a couple of people. Here again, the platform was strewn with utensils.

The first look at her future dwelling sent a shockwave through Nandini.

She couldn't believe her eyes. How could she live here?

At that very moment, another thought flashed her mind: *Did I make a mistake?*

She was in for more surprises as the day progressed. The house had a limited water supply, and they had to get buckets of water from the borewell in the compound which was two floors below. The toilet was common for all the residents of that floor. And of course, all the work in the house, which included the cooking, cleaning, and washing the utensils, had to be done by them. As she watched Rajan's mother performing these chores, it dawned upon her that they would also expect her to do the same.

That night, as she lay on the mattress spread on the floor of the kitchen, which was the only way they could get some privacy, tears of anguish and despair started rolling down her cheeks as she imagined herself performing the daily chores. For someone who had not even filled a glass of water herself, who assumed that the unlimited flow of water in her house was a natural entitlement, and who had never spent a night without the comfort of an air conditioner, the first day in her new house was a horrific experience.

*I have to tell Rajan that we have to move to a bigger house with decent facilities*, she thought.

The next morning, as Rajan was getting ready for work, Nandini broached the subject.

'Rajan, why don't we look for a bigger house to start our new life?' she asked.

'My dear Nandini,' he replied, 'a bigger house costs money. Right now, my salary is just enough to pay the EMIs for the loans that my father has taken. Once I start my new business, things will be very different.'

'But that will take time ...' She sighed. 'How can I live here?'

The last part came out inadvertently.

'I know it will be difficult initially, but you will adjust,' Rajan replied nonchalantly. 'I am getting late to work now. Just help my mother with the housework. Let us go out for dinner in the evening.'

A frustrated Nandini just couldn't get herself to do any housework. She lay there on the bed, all irritable and desperate for an escape.

At that very moment, there was a knock. Her father-in-law opened the door.

'Is this Rajan's house?' a man's deep-throated voice asked.

Nandini heard the voice and immediately recognised it.

She got up from the bed and walked to the door.

'Uncle,' she addressed the person standing there, 'please come in.'

Babu was one of the trusted aides of her father and one of his oldest employees. He was a like a family member.

'Nandu,' he said, 'what have you done? You could have at least discussed with me before taking such an important step. I would have spoken to your father. By running away, you have messed up everything. Your father is not only angry but also disappointed with you.'

Tears were flowing down her cheeks. She was not sure whether this outpouring of emotions was because of what Babu had said or a display of her innermost feelings in that moment.

'Don't worry, dear,' Babu continued. 'Nothing is lost. I will explain everything to your father. I have come to take you home. We will decide what to do along with your parents.'

This was a big moment for her. In her current state of mind, she wanted to jump at this opportunity. She looked around at Rajan's parents. They seemed to be anxiously waiting for a response.

Her mind was compelling her to go with Babu while her heart was still with Rajan. And her heart spoke that day.

'Uncle,' Nandini said slowly, 'I am married to Rajan now. I have to live with him. If you do want to help me, please convince my parents to accept this marriage.'

Babu looked around the room and then fixed his gaze on her.

'We can work out everything, but first you need to come home with me,' he insisted.

'I cannot do that, Uncle' she said and got up from the bed and went into the kitchen.

Babu stood up, looked at Rajan's parents, and left.

'Rajan,' Nandini said softly, 'I don't mean to hurt you. Please try to understand.'

Nandini and Rajan were having dinner at a restaurant that evening.

Rajan held her hand and said, 'Tell me.'

Nandini spoke. 'It's not my fault that I have lived in a house which had everything. I have not done any housework in my entire life. I can do anything for you, but it will take time for me to adjust to this new life. All I am saying is can we buy a bigger house? Maybe ... we can use some money from my account.'

Rajan looked into her eyes and said, 'Whatever you say, sweetheart. I am not keen on using your money for this, but I want to see you happy. I will pay back the money as soon as my new business starts prospering.'

'I am sure that will happen soon my dear,' Nandini assured him. 'I love you.'

Rajan thought for a moment and spoke. 'My dear, I have a plan but ...'

He stopped midsentence.

'Tell me, dear,' she urged.

'You know how passionate I am about my new business,' he said hesitantly. 'I have been trying to get some investors but have not been successful so far. I am beginning to lose hope, and that is frustrating. So, I was wondering if ...'

He paused again. But Nandini had read his mind.

'Why are you hesitating my dear?' she said. 'After all, the money in my account is for our better life. I am sure you will use it well.'

'Of course I will, my dear,' Rajan assured her. 'I don't know how to thank you for this. You are the best thing to have happened to me.'

The very next day, Rajan accompanied Nandini to the bank and helped her withdraw all the money in her account. He even mortgaged the gold against additional loans. He promised to share some good news very soon.

In a week's time, the couple moved into a rented two-bedroom apartment with Rajan's parents. Nandini was happy that she had a room for herself now. Some of her initial anxiety seemed to be over. That was until they had their first visitor.

'Appa … Amma …' Nandini screamed with joy, seeing her parents at the door one day.

Her father was staid as always, and her mother seemed as if she would break down any time. Rajan's parents greeted them, but her father ignored them, and her mother was forced to comply. Her father walked in and did not even bother to sit down. He went straight to the point.

'Nandini, you have been the apple of our eye. We have pampered you and given you everything you wanted. Probably, we were wrong. I have told you before as well. For me, nothing comes before our family honour. And you have brought our family into disrepute.'

Nandini had been expecting this encounter for some time now, but she would always imagine the conversation to be very different. She feared the worst now.

Her father continued his monologue.

'I was completely against it, but even I cannot come in the way of motherly love. I have decided to give you one more chance. Come home with us now, and we will forgive you for everything.'

'Appa!' Nandini cried in despair. 'Please don't do this to me. I love you very much. It was that love which forced me to take this step. I knew you will never agree to my marriage with Rajan. But I love him too and cannot dream of a life without him.'

'Nandini,' her father said without any emotions. 'Are you going to come with us or not?'

Her mother was crying now and intervened 'Nandu dear, I beg of you to come with us. We will find a nice groom for you. You will be very happy.'

'Amma!' Nandini exclaimed as she went and embraced her mother. She started sobbing uncontrollably and her mother reciprocated.

After a few minutes, Nandini spoke again 'Amma, how can you say this? I am now married to Rajan. Please accept him. He is a nice man. His parents are so nice. They treat me like their daughter ... Amma ... please.'

Before her mother could say anything, her father intervened loudly.

'Nandini, I want your decision now.'

'Appa ... please,' she cried, falling at her father's feet.

Her father moved away as she fell on the ground and continued crying hysterically.

Her father was getting even more impatient.

'Nandini, what's your decision?'

She looked up from where she was sitting and folded her hands in desperation. 'Appa, I cannot leave Rajan. Please understand,' she said amid the flood of tears.

A visibly angry father declared loudly 'In that case, you are dead as far as we are concerned. I disown you.'

'Appa ... no,' Nandini wailed.

Her shocked mother was now bawling but was unable to say anything in defiance of her husband. Rajan's parents, who were mute spectators to this family drama, stepped forward to help.

'Sir,' Rajan's father said, 'I know this is your family matter, but you are taking a very harsh decision. Please think about it.'

Her father looked at him and responded, 'I hold you equally responsible for this situation, but I don't want to say anything to you in your home. That does not mean I will just hear you. I don't need your advice.' Looking at his wife, he said, 'Come, let's leave. I will think that we have only two daughters now,' and he made a move to the door.

'Appa,' Nandini got up and ran to her father and hugged his back 'I am sorry for all this. But please try and understand. I will be happy only if you accept my marriage.'

'Laxmi!' he bellowed. 'Are you coming now, or should I leave you here as well?'

Her father left the house, and his wife followed him without saying an additional word, leaving behind a wailing Nandini and her shocked parents-in-law.

Nandini had lived a life of entitlement. Her fascination with movies and the *reel life* of characters had probably drawn her to a man who was probably in love with her but was very different from her in every respect. Her love and trust for him was so much more than her family ties and the wealth that came with it.

However, this very sign of blind trust was the beginning of the worst time of her life.

# 7

'Why did you take such a hasty decision?' Rajan admonished her when he came home that evening and heard about the day's emotional encounter.

Nandini did not expect this response from her husband and retorted, 'What do you mean, Rajan?'

'I mean your father has disowned you. Do you even understand what it means? You will not get a share of his wealth,' he asked in anger.

'What are you saying, Rajan? I did not know that my father's wealth was so important for you,' she quizzed him.

'I mean ... don't you want to lead a good life?' he tried to explain.

'Can't you give me a good life, Rajan? I don't need my father's wealth,' she asserted.

Rajan was visibly agitated and replied, 'Don't be crazy, Nandini. You have been cribbing for a bigger house. You have been complaining about the housework you have to do. This is just the beginning. My business needs a lot of money. Where will we get that?'

'I don't believe it, Rajan. So, what should I have done?' a livid Nandini asked.

He shouted, 'You should have gone home with your parents. Once they cooled down, you could have made them understand. Now you have removed all chances of a reconciliation.'

With that, he threw the glass of water that he was holding on the ground and left the house in a hush.

From that day onwards, his behaviour towards her turned on its head. He ignored her presence in the house, and any attempt by her to talk to him was met with verbal and physical abuse. This continued for many days. She considered going back to her parents' house many times but could not muster the courage to face her father. She had nowhere to go, and with every passing day, Nandini went into a severe state of depression. From a carefree girl who had vivid dreams in her eyes, she slipped into a state where nothing mattered.

As if the struggles with her own life were not enough, she had the misfortune of bringing another into this world. Nine months after their hurried decision to spend their life together, Nandini delivered a baby boy. Her pregnancy was very complicated, and the doctor ruled out the possibility of an abortion. Nandini was hardly in a mental state even to take care of herself, and it was Rajan's parents who donned the role of foster parents to little Bala.

Rajan's behaviour oscillated from the very violent to the caring husband, the latter mostly to satisfy his primal desires. He would keep pushing her to go to her parents' house and demand her share of the property. She refused vehemently, which led to further abuse and alienation. He even tried to hire a lawyer to fight her case, but her father's position in society made it difficult to find one. Desperation made him hit the bottle. His performance in the company dropped, but his skills and previous performances helped him stay in the good books of his bosses. His business was nowhere near taking off. Without the necessary focus and with burgeoning debts, it slipped further into losses.

Bala was a restless child, constantly needing attention. He would not remain still even for a moment and it was extremely tough on Rajan's parents to manage him, as they themselves were not getting any younger. Rajan and Nandini's involvement in Bala's life would be intermittent—he when there was nothing else to do and she on the days when her depression could be controlled. As Bala grew up into a toddler, he started having extreme mood swings. He would be hyperactive on some days and completely in his shell on other days.

Just when all seemed lost for this family, Rajan's boss offered him a posting in Singapore. His boss had been seeing his performance deteriorate and had made enquiries. He realised that the root cause was the problems in his personal life, especially his troubled relationship with his wife. The Singapore posting required someone with Rajan's skill, and his boss also realised that having more time for each other would bring Rajan closer to his wife. Rajan's parents were too old to travel anyway.

Rajan, Nandini, and Bala travelled to Singapore to begin a new life.

## 8

My assistant, Sandra, buzzed me on my intercom.

'Hello, ma'am. Miss Irene is here to meet you,' she said in her pleasant voice.

'Please send her in,' I replied.

Irene was a teacher at National Talent Preschool. I had met her at a social event, and her pleasing personality endeared her to me. She was instrumental in inviting me to her school a couple of months ago to have an interactive session on child psychology with the teachers. I was pleasantly surprised with her sudden appearance at my clinic.

'May I come in, Doctor?' she asked as she poked her head into my room.

'Of course you can, Irene,' I said and walked to the door to greet her. 'How are you, Irene?' I asked.

'Very good, Doctor, and you look very good as always,' she said with a smile.

She had this knack of making people feel good with her positive comments. For some reason, she had always referred to me as 'Doctor', and today was no different. After the initial pleasantries, she came to the subject that had brought her here.

'I am here to talk to you about a child in my school. He is otherwise a good kid but, on most days, he tends to be extremely hyperactive. On other days, he tends to be silent and remains aloof from everybody.'

I was listening and also silently admiring this young lady for taking the extra efforts beyond her normal call of duty.

She continued, 'It was my duty to inform his parents about this behaviour. I invited them to the school. They did not turn up, so I invited them again. When they did not come for the second time, I decided to visit their home. In a very short time, I realised that this was a dysfunctional family. The mother seemed to be highly depressed. The father was aggressive and blamed the school for his behaviour. I am more concerned about the child, and I therefore suggested that they should take the child for therapy. I was surprised when they accepted my suggestion. I have given them your details so I thought I will give you the background.'

I said, 'Thank you Irene for taking these efforts. This is highly commendable. I will wait for their visit and see what needs to be done. What is the child's name?'

'Bala Rajan,' she replied.

Sure enough after a week, Bala was brought to the clinic by his parents.

'He doesn't sit still. He always wants to go to the toilet. He scribbles on the wall with his crayons. He sleeps only for a couple of hours. He is very moody. We have received reports from his school that he gets aggressive with other children …'

Bala's father Rajan shared a long list of complaints.

All along, I was watching the boy. He was seated in front of me, but his eyes were moving all over the room. He would scratch his head, get down from the chair, get up again, and fiddle with something on the table. When his father called out his name, he would be still for a brief moment and then start his routine again. I also noticed that the mother hardly said anything. She had this forlorn look. She seemed to be so much older than her husband, overweight and seemingly unconcerned about the subject of discussion.

I tried to elicit a response from her.

'Mrs Rajan, what are your observations?'

She searched for an answer and said, 'The same that my husband has described,' she said, and she was silent again. I was sure she had more to say. Her face suggested that.

I addressed the child.

'Bala! would you like to do some colouring?' I asked softly.

His face brightened, but he did not answer.

I called Sandra and asked her to get some crayons and papers from the adjacent room.

I laid them on the table and asked Bala to do some colouring for me. He was onto it immediately.

I understood from Mr Rajan that he was working for an IT company and his wife, Nandini, was a housewife. She had been ill lately, which explained her aloof behaviour. He affirmed that he was a good father and that the child might have some disorders which needed to be corrected.

I heard him out.

After a while, Bala lifted the sheet of paper and showed it around proudly.

'Bravo!' I exclaimed. 'You were very fast. Please show me what you have done.'

That acknowledgement enthused him to bring the sheet of paper to me. He tried to explain, 'This is a house. This is a boy. This is a playground. This is a policeman.'

'That's wonderful Bala,' I said. 'I want you to come here regularly and do more drawings for me. I will have a candy with me next time. Will you come?'

He nodded.

All through this interaction, the parents seemed disinterested.

'Mr Rajan,' I said, 'Bala needs an outlet for his nervous energy. Buy him more drawing books and encourage him to colour. Enrol him in a swimming class or athletics class, which will help in expending his physical energy. Is that possible?'

'Yes, ma'am,' he confirmed. 'Anything to make him calmer.'

'Would you like to say anything, Mrs Rajan?' I asked the mother.

'Nothing' was her monotone response.

We mutually agreed to have a few more sessions.

Both the parents came with Bala for the next few sessions. In every session, I applied the win-win method asking him to draw, create clay models, or build something using Lego. He would create many different scenes, but there was one constant in all his drawings, clay models, and structures built with Lego.

There would always be a policeman.

Even in a drawing of what he said was a school, there was a policeman. In his clay models, there would be a figure wearing a cap.

'What is this fixation on a policeman?' I asked Rajan during one of the sessions.

He had no answer. Neither did his mother.

'Bala, what is this policeman doing?' I asked him.

He looked around and did not answer In spite of some prodding. I had to find out. I also had to get his mother to talk.

I got both these opportunities in the next session.


Nandini and Bala walked into my clinic that day without Rajan.

Even at first sight, I could see them being visibly less anxious. Nandini actually greeted me, which she had never done before.

'Where is Mr Rajan?' I asked.

'He had some important meeting,' Nandini replied.

I gave the Lego pieces to Bala and asked him to build something for me. While he was busy with the colourful pieces of Lego, I initiated a conversation with Nandini.

'Who are you?' I asked.

She was startled with the question and stared blankly.

I repeated the question.

'His mother,' she said, pointing to Bala.

'Good. What else?' I continued.

'I am also a wife,' she said.

'Good ... tell me more. Who are you?'

She thought about the question and looked up with tears in her eyes.

'Nandini.' I held her hand, 'I want to know only about the person Nandini today. Can I get to know her?'

I remained silent and gave her the space that she yearned for.

'I have nothing to say,' she said after some thought.

I prompted her, 'I am sure Nandini was born somewhere, she grew up somewhere, she had a family before she got married, had a married life, and so on. I want to hear all of this from you.'

It took a while, but she finally opened up. She continued uninterrupted for close to an hour, during which time I seemed to be nonexistent. She oscillated between the heights of ecstasy to the depths of despair and her life seemed like a rollercoaster ride. Her narration was interspersed with tears, silence, screams, and even the rare smile.

When she finished her narration, she heaved a sigh of relief as the many years of bottled up emotions were finally let out.

For me, the story of her life reignited my thoughts on the vagaries of life.

Nandini was born with a silver spoon, but she squandered it all to be with the love of her life. The object of her love was equally besotted, but not with her. He saw her wealth as the best way to fulfil his business aspirations. Nandini's running away from home was well planned but what he did not plan for, was the extreme reaction of her parents in disowning her. Without her wealth, Nandini meant nothing to him. She was now an object of scorn and bore the brunt of his frustrations. The unintended arrival of the baby made matters worse.

In the society they lived in, divorce was a rarity, and to get divorced with a child was almost blasphemous. For her parents, the baby also effectively ended any chance of getting her marriage annulled. Nandini was unable to cope with

Rajan's betrayal and her parents' extreme action to disown her, and she slowly slipped into a state of depression. I would also attribute her mental state to the feeling of utter disgust at her own decisions. She was probably in a state of mind where she could not even trust herself.

Very importantly, she slipped into a state of depression during her pregnancy. Would that be an influence on Bala's personality? This was an eye-opener for me. It is a well-known fact that the environment during his growing-up years influence an individual's belief systems and behaviour patterns. Bala was a testament to the fact that the environment can even influence a foetus.

As I reflected on Nandini's story, little Bala shouted from where he was seated.

'See my zoo,' he said excitedly.

I went up to him and surveyed his creation. He had arranged many Lego pieces which appeared to be animals behind a set of barriers which seemed to be a fence. As I admired his creativity, one particular object caught my eye.

'Who is this Bala?' I asked.

'This is Bala,' he said with pride.

'What is he wearing?' I enquired.

'Bala is a policeman,' he replied.

'That's wonderful, Bala,' I said and encouraged him. 'Bala will be a good policeman. Oh! I see the policeman also had a gun in his hand.'

'Yes,' he continued, 'Bala will put all robbers in jail.'

'Who is this?' I asked, pointing to another figure of a man.

'Appa,' he said.

'Oh!' I exclaimed. 'What is he doing in the zoo?'

'He is a robber, and Bala will put him in jail,' he asserted.

'Why, Bala?' I asked, wanting to continue this conversation. 'What did he do?'

'He scolds me and beats Amma,' he said nonchalantly.

I was taken aback by this rather innocent comment, which had a profound meaning.

All this while, Bala had been expressing his fears through the drawings and Lego creations. In the fictional world that he was creating, he was always the policeman who would reprimand the robber, who symbolised his father.

I looked at Nandini as if to tell her, 'Did you hear that? This is the effect of the parents' behaviour on their child.'

It was a day of revelations. The absence of Rajan had turned into a boon. The many pieces of the jigsaw puzzle were falling into place. I needed to now focus on the remedy.

## 9

During the next few sessions, I had some tough discussions with Rajan and Nandini.

'Mr and Mrs Rajan,' I stated. 'Your child, Bala, has bipolar disorder.'

'What?' Rajan exclaimed 'What is that?'

I explained 'Bipolar disorder is a mental illness marked by extreme mood swings from high to low and from low to high. Highs are periods of mania, while lows are periods of depression. The mood swings may even become mixed, so you might feel elated and depressed at the same time.'

'How did it happen?' Rajan asked.

'There could be many reasons. Some genetic, some acquired,' I explained.

'What is the cure?' Rajan enquired.

'Bipolar disorder is a mental illness,' I explained. 'Of course, it can be cured, but like every mental illness, it requires the cooperation of the individual and the people around him. Both of you are also part of his cure.'

Rajan looked at his wife and then at me. 'It's very difficult to manage him. We will do as you suggest.'

I stated, 'I will need to have separate sessions with both of you. From the next session, I want Mrs Rajan to come with Bala for a few sessions followed by a few sessions with you, Mr Rajan.'

'OK,' Rajan said, and his wife nodded.

The next few sessions with Nandini were intense. I helped her trace back the events in her life, the decisions she had made, and the consequences. I helped her see the importance of maintaining relationships and how the lack of it would affect someone. I helped her come to terms with where she was in life now and motivated her to plan for a better future. Very importantly, I convinced her to attempt a reconciliation with her parents. I told Nandini in so many words that her inability to manage her own life was affecting their child, that her stress and anxieties were being transferred to the child.

I was attempting to provide her with a fresh start.

I had separate sessions with Rajan where I made an attempt to make him realise that his misdemeanours had severely affected two lives. For someone with a big ego, he could not easily accept any responsibility for their current situation. He had created a self-image of being strong and always right. I had to break through that barrier and help him see the futility of his actions, which had resulted in his own life getting derailed. He had to change if he wanted his own life to be better, and that change would positively affect the people around him. Over multiple sessions, I correlated his actions and behaviours to the mental condition of Nandini and that of his child.

Finally, he broke down.

He reflected on the many wrong decisions that he had taken at various stages. He admitted that he was blinded by his obsession to make money and had seen Nandini as a conduit. He did feel sorry for her, but the greed for money and riches overshadowed any feeling of compassion that he may have harboured. Somewhere deep in his unconscious mind, he had attributed all the failures in his life to Nandini.

When I shared the policeman story with him, he couldn't control his tears.

'I am a total failure,' he cried. 'I have not been a good son, a good husband, or even a good father.'

I counselled him to start creating a bond with his child. I suggested that he should have conversations with Bala and have more exclusive father-son time with him. I made him realise that he needs to change his behaviour towards his parents and wife. He needs to ensure that this change was visible to Bala, as this would indirectly change his perceptions about family and relationships.

Once the individual sessions had started taking effect, I focussed on some marriage counselling sessions. They had to decide on their relationship for their own sake since their life and that of their child hinged on it. The individual sessions had created a shift in their outlook, which helped in the discussions about their marriage.

I spent the maximum amount of time with Bala. Here was a child who had not seen love. He was living a life of fear and anxiety and unable to come to terms with them. I employed the win-win situation (situation by which group participation leads to all participants benefits) and engaged him in a lot of games using cards, lego, colouring, and human faces. I worked on improving his concentration through attention-span activities. I would make him sit in one place for five minutes with the incentive of a reward. Gradually, I increased it to ten minutes and after many months managed to make him sit still for a period of thirty minutes. I did activities with him in the park and other places of his interest, like the zoo and bird park. I visited his school from time to time and had conversations with Irene. It was heartening to see the positive effect of all these sessions through Irene's feedback. At the start of a new academic year, Bala was enrolled in a new school. After the initial period of anxiety, he coped well with the new environment and seemed much more settled there.

It has been more than two years since I started my sessions with Rajan, Nandini, and Bala. They are now a happier family. With his personal life more settled, Rajan's performance at work improved. Nandini is more assured of herself. Her attempts at reaching out to her parents have at least put them on talking terms. Bala is more focussed now. His attention span is better. He is more attentive, and his drawings don't have a policeman anymore.

This story had a happy ending after all—just like the movies.

# 10

The world of movies is a make-believe world, created for our entertainment. The characters in most commercial movies are larger than life and are able to perform super-human activities in fictitiously created situations.

When the audience watches these movies, they are transported to a different world, where they see themselves in the characters on screen. Their own struggles are forgotten as they live this *reel life* for the three hours. The problem starts when we don't come out of this character even after the movie ends. We imbibe a number of the character traits and expect others to have similar exaggerated traits without realising that this is not humanly possible.

Nandini was one such person who carried the characters home with her. The situations which led to her falling in love with Rajan were very much larger than life and fit perfectly into her virtual view of the world. The decisions that she took were immature, without enough thought on the future. How could she not even see the home of the person she loved, the place where she was expected to live a large part of her life? How could she be so blinded by her love to disregard her own family, for whom she was a favourite child? How could she be so naive to give off all her wealth to Rajan without any thought of her own future? Was she responsible for her condition?

Nandini's parents must have loved her, but were they right in imposing marriage upon her without her consent? Would Nandini have taken the drastic step of running away if her parents had been more open? Nandini did make a big mistake by eloping with Rajan, but they were adults, after all. Was her parents' decision to disown Nandini justified?

Rajan's parents were mute spectators to the whole episode being played out in front of them. They supported Nandini's lack of experience in housework and also showered their love and attention on little Bala. Could they have exerted some influence on their son and changed his behaviour?

Was Rajan the villain of this story? He was born in a poor family but was ambitious. He made the best use of the opportunity to get educated and acquire a decent qualification which would have provided him a secure life. Why did he succumb to the lure of turning rich overnight? Did he decide to court Nandini only for her riches? Can your ambition be so powerful as to disregard every other emotion? He was sure that Nandini's family would never accept him and plotted the elopement with Nandini. When his subsequent plan of her family accepting their marriage eventually fell through, was he right in rejecting Nandini? Even when their child came into this world, was it not a good enough reason for him to stop blaming Nandini for his unfulfilled desires.

And finally, what about Bala? He had his entire life in front of him. He was brought into this world with a disadvantage, and the negatives continued to pile up even after he was born. Why should a child bear the consequences of their parents' misdeeds?

I wish the generation of today take informed decisions when it comes to choosing their life partners. It is not only their life but the lives of their parents and their future child that is at stake.

# CHAPTER 9

# THE GREED

## 1

The buzzing sound of the mobile phone woke him up from a deep slumber.

He tried to find his bearings in the darkness, and it took a while before he realised that it was not a dream. His head was aching, and the sound of the phone was only making it worse.

He hastily moved his hand in the direction of the lamp next to his bed and switched it on. It had been a while since he had decided to keep his mobile phone away from the bed, what with all the talk of radiation and its ill effects. He had even made it a habit to switch off the ringer and turn on the vibration mode, but his passive mind seemed to be alert to even this sound.

John Houghton was a British citizen and had been working in Singapore for close to five years now. He was the high-profile CEO of Mobitrax, a mobile phone company which had a manufacturing base in China but assembly centres in many Southeast Asian countries. The year was 2008 and mobile telephony was beginning to change the way the world was doing business. With more countries around the world enhancing their telecommunications network, the demand for mobile phones was increasing exponentially. Mobitrax was founded in 2001 and had grown to more than two thousand employees within a few years. Touted as the pioneer in low-cost high-resolution camera phones, the company was among the top three brands sold in Southeast Asia.

John was a shark to the core and revelled at the opportunity offered to him by the promoters of Mobitrax to turn the company around from the verge of bankruptcy to making a profit.

'I accept the challenge,' he stated animatedly when the promoters appraised him about the current issues ailing the company.

Of course, the big bonus laid out as bait would have been too good to resist, but for John, the mountain that he had to climb seemed more appealing than the big bucks on offer.

That was three years ago. As soon as the contract terms were finalised, he got down to business. Ruthless cost-cutting measures were interspersed with strategically planned media campaigns, and within a year, the company was breaking even. Many people lost their jobs in the tsunami that hit Mobitrax, but for John, emotions had no role to play in the corporate boardroom. There were many ex-employees who went to court, but John had preempted this possibility and had created a very strong legal team which managed these matters well while not allowing any damage to the brand's reputation.

Last night was the launch event of a new model from their flagship Lunar series. The prelaunch media blitz had already created a buzz among teenagers, and sales were expected to hit the roof. Many Hollywood celebrities were special invitees to the event, which was covered by most of the business media. The party went on well into the night, and John had hit the bed in a drunken state only at 4 a.m.

The mobile phone continued to vibrate as John slowly made his way to the study table and picked it up. The number on the screen was not in his contacts, which irritated him more. Even while his mind was telling him to ignore the call, he inadvertently picked up the phone. A voice that did not seem familiar was on the line.

'Hello,' John said groggily.

'Hello,' whispered the husky voice.

'Who is this?' an irritated John asked as the headache was making him uncomfortable.

'It doesn't matter who I am,' the person continued. 'What matters is the information I am going to give you.'

The rather intriguing statement made him alert.

'Who is this?' John asked again with more purpose.

'You pride yourself on your high-quality standards, don't you?' the person at the other end said with a smirk. 'You think you are the only person who works hard in the company. Let me tell you how inefficient you and your company processes are.'

John's eyes fell on his watch. It was 5:03 a.m., hardly the time for a discussion on his company standards.

'What the hell are you talking about?' he growled in anger.

'You obstinate,' the person responded haughtily. 'Learn to listen to others.'

John was taken aback by the unparliamentary language and arrogance in the voice. He remained silent.

'I have some information with me that proves how useless your standards are.'

'What are you talking about?' John retorted, unable to hold himself back.

'You heard it right,' the man continued. 'Someone is taking out a mobile phone from your company every day, and no one cares a damn about it. This news will be in the press by tomorrow morning. You will have no place to hide. Your company will be bankrupt very soon.'

Even as he was listening, John's sharp mind had started thinking about what was being said. He was not used to hearing such a level of verbal abuse, definitely not at five in the morning.

Just as John was about to respond, the person shouted, 'go to the devil you,' and disconnected the phone. The conversation ended as abruptly as it had begun.

John looked at his watch again. It was 5:14 a.m. Still too early for a normal person, but for John, as in the mood as he was in, the time of the day did not matter. It never had.

He made a call to his legal head, who was used to getting calls from John at odd hours and discussed possibilities. He asked his good connections at the telecom service provider to dig into the source of the call. He called his communications head and asked him to take care of the media side of things. Within the next thirty minutes, the sleepy-eyed leadership team of Mobitrax were on a mission.

## 2

Yang Mi was your typical Singaporean woman, managing a corporate career and a family, which included her husband (Deng Xiao) and two schoolgoing kids. Her day would begin very early, at 5 a.m., getting the kids ready for school, preparing breakfast for herself and her husband, giving instructions to the maid, getting ready, and travelling to work. As the IT manager at Mobitrax, she had significant responsibilities at work which required many late sittings. Back home, she would spend time with her kids, helping them with their studies before tucking them in their beds. Somewhere around 10pm is when she would have some time for herself and a conversation with her husband before her eyes would shut off on their own.

Yang Mi was lucky to have a supportive husband who helped her with the household chores, but his job required him to travel most days of the month.

Life was moving in the fast lane, and even her vacations were a blur. In short, she was leading the life of an average Singaporean.

Like most others, Yang Mi had a dream. She wanted to travel around the world, live in expensive hotels, and splurge on shopping. But unlike most others, for whom it was a passing fantasy, for Yang Mi, it was an obsession.

Whenever she would get some free time during her busy schedule, she would be reading travelogues, watching videos of exotic holiday destinations, and browsing through the catalogue of famous fashion brands. She had an opportunity to travel to Japan for a business conference recently, and during the entire trip, she was like a kid visiting Disneyland for the first time. She would work her socks off to become eligible for the annual performance bonus, which took her one small step towards her goal. As a result of the many years of hard work, they were able to save some decent money from their monthly family income.

Her aging windowed mother lived nearby and was independent—up until this point.

Her mother had been complaining of uneasiness for some days, and Yang Mi accompanied her to Holy Cross Hospital for a routine check-up. After she underwent the standard tests, Yang Mi and her mother met the GP for the reports. One look at the GP and Yang Mi knew something was wrong.

'I would recommend some more tests for your mother,' the GP said rather pensively.

A concerned Yang Mi asked, 'What's the matter, Doctor?'

'I can't say anything until I am certain,' he explained. 'But I would really recommend these tests.'

He went on to explain the tests and took their consent. The reports were expected after a couple of days. They were given an appointment with the specialist doctor from the oncology department.

'I am afraid', the doctor at the Holy Cross Hospital revealed after studying the stack of reports in front of her, 'your mother has cancer.'

Yang Mi could not believe her ears.

'Are you sure, Doctor?' she enquired with a deep sense of apprehension.

The doctor explained, 'The reports are suggesting second-stage cancer, which is curable.'

Yang Mi was devastated, but she took her mother's hand in hers and held it tightly to let her know that she was being strong.

'What do you suggest now?' a concerned Yang Mi asked the doctor.

The doctor replied, 'Since the cancer has metastasised beyond her breasts, we will start a few sessions of chemotherapy and radiation apart from a course of medication. After three months, we will know whether we need to perform surgery.'

Yang Mi tried hard to control her tears as she thought of the rather painful treatment that her mother would have to go through.

'And ...?' She hesitated, wanting to ask, 'What are the chances, Doctor?'

The doctor, who had handled many patients before, seemed to read her mind. 'There is a very good chance of recovery, but the process will be slow.'

He looked at Yang Mi's mother and continued, 'You have to be patient, Mrs Wei. You have to remain positive. Keep your spirits high. I would even recommend some counselling for you.'

That evening, Yang Mi and Deng Xiao had a long chat with her mother. They explained the treatment and assured her of their support. Yang Mi was happy that her mother was reasonably positive about the whole thing.

If Yang Mi's life was hectic until then, it became crazy now.

Apart from her other routine, she had to accompany her mother to the hospital every week and also spend more time with her almost every day.

As the treatment progressed, the medical expenses started mounting. The tests done after three months revealed further complications. The hospital visits increased, and so did the bills. While Yang Mi loved her mother and would do anything for her, the pressures of the job, the stress of managing the home, the sight of her mother's failing health, and the financial strain were all taking a toll on her health. Many sleepless nights, a nonexistent appetite, and high blood pressure only made it worse.

Something had to be done to turnaround this spiral, and an unintended mistake showed the way.

## 3

Mobitrax had implemented stringent quality standards, which it highlighted as a USP but with pressure from sales to constantly increase the speed to market, compromises were becoming the norm rather than an exception.

Yang Mi was the IT manager at Mobitrax, and her team maintained the ERP systems, which churned out terabytes of data every day. Her team created the automated reports, which would form the basis for management decision-making. As a part of her routine, she would randomly reconcile the reports with actual data to verify their authenticity. During one such reconciliation exercise, a discrepancy caught her eye. The physical count of the P6 models did not tally with the online report. She ran some queries on the database and realised that this discrepancy had been in existence for more than a couple of months but had not come to light. The actual count of the P6 mobile phones would always be one more than what the online report suggested. She checked the manual inventory report maintained by the final dispatch team at the warehouse, and it confirmed this discrepancy. She was surprised that no one had noticed this difference. Probably, the number was too small to be of concern.

That evening, as she was returning back from work, a vague thought emerged. She mulled over it through the night and dismissed it as nonsensical. As she went about her daily chores and sought a release to her pent-up stress, the thought kept coming back to her. In a moment of deep frustration, she decided to put her thought into action the very next day.

She visited the finished goods section of their warehouse where the packed mobile phones were awaiting dispatch. As per the documented procedure, an operator in this section would take a physical count of all the phones being dispatched and update the daily inventory in the system. This data would then get uploaded on the server every night. Many programs would run during the night and a 'daily inventory summary' would be sent to the production head and the 'stock available for sale' would be sent to the head of sales every morning. This would form the basis for his sales plans.

Yang Mi had identified that while the operator seemed to be entering the physical count for the P6 model correctly, the count shown in the 'stock available for sale' report was one less than the actual number. Clearly, this was a programming error and would be easy to fix.

Yang Mi, however, had other ideas.

Yang Mi made her way through the many racks, full of packed boxes and at one particular section which she was sure was hidden from the CCTV cameras, she picked up a packed P6 phone, stuck a Velcro strip to it, and shoved it under her skirt. She had stuck some more Velcro strips between her legs and the two Velcro strips stuck to each other. She casually walked to the computer terminal, browsed some screens, and then silently walked out of the room. Her position in the company gave her access to the warehouse, and so the security guards at the entrance to this section did not stop her.

That evening, she drove to a part of the city which had a reputation for selling first copies of branded goods at throwaway prices. She spoke to a few store owners and finally met a lady in the bylanes behind the famous Mustafa market. The lady was ready to buy the P6 phone at a good price. She was also ready to buy more quantities from her in future.

She spent a nervous night tossing and turning in her bed. The first thing she did when she reached office was to check the P6 'Daily Inventory Summary' and the 'Stock available for Sale' reports. Since, she had taken away one phone, both the reports now showed the same number.

No one had noticed the difference between one phone earlier. Her unethical action had ensured that the reports now tallied so there was no reason for anyone to suspect that something had been wrong.

Yang Mi treaded cautiously the next day, slightly disturbed by her own actions. However, the money that she made from that act was significant and the possibility of being able to do this more often suppressed the muted feelings of apprehension.

An error in the system had given her an unintended lifeline, albeit unethically.

She would follow this routine initially every two days, but with the passage of time and an increase in her own confidence, this became a daily activity. In the race to achieve their own targets, no one in the company noticed this manipulation.

This went on for more than six months. Yang Mi was earning good money which was more than making up for the expenses of her mother's treatment. Her zest for life was restored.

### 4

'I pronounce you guilty,' the judge said.

'Please don't put me behind bars,' she started screaming. 'I have not done anything. I have to take care of my children. My old mother is suffering and needs me ... Please ... I beg of you.'

Everyone in the courtroom was shouting, 'Shame, shame, shame.'

She put her hands over her ears and violently shook her head, yelling, 'No ... no ... no.'

Yang Mi woke up abruptly from her sleep. She looked around and realised that she was in her own home. She was sweating profusely. She got out of bed, went into the kitchen, and had a glass of cold water. She was feeling suffocated. She stepped out of the house, slowly closing the door behind her. She took the elevator to the bottom floor and stepped out of the apartment. She felt better as soon as she was able to breathe the fresh air. There was a slight breeze blowing, and there was a definite chill in the cool January air. She tilted her head to the sky and soaked in as much of it. Slowly, when she seemed in control, Yang Mi started a slow walk around the apartment block, pondering over the dream.

*Am I doing the right thing?* she wondered. *What if I get caught? I will be in prison for many years. The risk is too high.*

But then a counterthought also made its appearance. *Why would I get caught? No one has any idea about my act. Even if I do get caught, they will only catch me with one phone. They will never be able to track the loss of the other phones.*

As she veered between these two extreme possibilities, the moral side of her came up with a solution.

She went back home and caught up on her sleep.

The next day, a little after lunch, she stepped outside her office, walked to the nearest telephone booth, and dialled a number.

'Hello! Felicia Chin speaking,' a sweet voice answered.

Miss Felicia Chin was the HR manager at Mobitrax.

'Hello, ma'am,' Yang Mi said. 'I would like to report something.'

'May I know who is speaking,' Ms Chin enquired politely.

'I cannot tell you that,' Yang Mi retorted, 'but I have some important information for you.'

There was silence, and then Ms Chin spoke.

'OK,' she said, 'tell me.'

'Someone is taking out a mobile phone from your warehouse every day. Your processes need to be tightened—'

'What are you saying?' Ms Chin interrupted. 'I want to know who you are.'

'I cannot tell you that,' Yang Mi responded firmly and disconnected the call.

Yang Mi casually walked back to the office and continued with her work.

She was hoping for some drastic measures to be put in place and some investigations to happen, but to her surprise, there were none.

Her mother's health was not getting any better. Multiple chemotherapy and radiation sessions had taken a toll on her mother's psyche, and her will to fight was not as pronounced as it was when the disease was detected almost a year ago. Yang Mi was required to spend more time with her. For someone who was going through a rather uneventful phase in her career, raising the spirits of someone else was not an easy task. She was living a kind of dual personality who would be motivating her mother to look at the beauty of life on one hand while herself needing someone who could lift her spirits. To make matters worse, her husband's travels also increased, and there was no one she could fall back on. The frustration welling inside her would burst out on her children, her maid, her colleagues at work, and even the shopkeepers. Some days would be so mentally tiring that even the pills she had started consuming did not work and she had to cry herself to sleep.

Back at work, her call to the HR head did not seem to have triggered any action.

With every passing day, her immoral side started speaking up. 'I told you so. They don't care.'

Just a few weeks after the bad dream, Yang Mi was back to taking the phones out of the warehouse. That year was a very good year for Mobitrax. The company had forayed into a few more countries, and sales was picking up everywhere. The city was littered with billboards showing the company's brand ambassador, a lovely Singaporean movie star holding a Mobitrax phone. That night as Yang Mi was watching television and a Mobitrax advertisement flashed on the screen, her husband commented.

'You are lucky to be working in such a wonderful company,' he said in admiration.

Yang Mi smiled and nodded her head in acknowledgement, but her mind began to wander again.

'Are they really good? If so, they should have done something about my call … maybe I called the wrong person … yes, maybe I called the wrong person.'

The next morning, she walked up to the phone booth again and called the company board line. When the operator answered, she asked for Mr Irfan Mohammed, the warehouse manager.

'Hello,' Mr Mohammed answered in a baritone which Yang Mi was familiar with.

'Hello, Mr Mohammed,' she said, almost lowering her voice to a whisper. 'Listen to me carefully.'

There was silence, which suggested that Mr Mohammed was listening. She continued.

'I would like to warn you that someone is stealing mobile phones from the warehouse,' she stated.

There was a sound of laughter.

'This is the best joke I have heard for many days,' Mr Mohammed quipped in between the guffaws. 'Who are you anyway?'

'I cannot tell you that, but you got to believe me,' Yang Mi said, trying to sound as convincing as possible, 'what I am saying is true.'

'Listen lady,' the warehouse manager said in a more serious tone, 'if you are making fun of me, let it stop you right here. I don't like to talk to strangers anyway.'

'Why don't you understand?' she persisted. 'My identity is not important. Please try and understand what I am—'

Mr Mohammed interrupted her. 'Lady,' he said sternly, 'I am on my way for my *namaaz*! I don't have time for your nonsense.'

Another call had ended abruptly. Another attempt to close the doors on her, now uncontrollable, habit seemed to have failed.

Nothing seemed to have changed in Mobitrax. Everyone was busy with work and meeting their deadlines. Like Ms Felicia Chin, Mr Mohammed also seemed to have ignored Yang Mi's call.

While the mobile phones were bringing in good money, Yang Mi's conscience continued to prick her from time to time. However, she had gotten so deep into the act, and the rewards were so high that she was not able to get rid of the habit voluntarily. Whether she wanted to come out of the habit was also in question.

When she could no longer bear this constant tussle with the moral side of her, she decided to make one last attempt. This time, she wanted to be sure that the person she would call would take some action and deny her access to the phones. She tossed and turned through the night. Just before the break of dawn, she walked out of the house to a phone booth nearby and made the call—the call which she believed would change her life.

It did, but not in the way that she had planned.

## 5

I had just returned from my morning jog when my phone rang.

'Dr Pandit,' the caller said, 'I am Officer Chen Lun from the police department. We need your assistance.'

'Officer,' I asked, surprised at being called so early in the morning, 'what is this about?'

'Dr Pandit, I request you to come to the office of Mobitrax. I will explain everything when you are here.'

'Mobitrax?' I asked as the brand's prominent logo danced in front of my eyes.

'Yes, Dr Pandit,' said the officer and shared the address.

'When do you want me to come there?' I enquired.

'Right away, Doctor,' the officer requested.

I do get calls from clients at odd hours, as some of them live in a different country, but getting a call from the police was a rarity.

Not wanting to get mired in any kind of speculations, I got ready and reached Mobitrax office by 9 a.m. A lady received me and requested me to accompany her. As I followed her inside the office, I was surprised by the presence of so many police officers there. We soon reached a door with a sign 'CEO' on it.

When I entered the room, a police officer stepped forward and greeted me, 'Hello, Dr Pandit. I am Officer Chen Lun. I called you today.'

'Hello, Officer,' I acknowledged his greeting and looked around the room.

The gentleman behind the desk rose and came forward to shake my hand. In a strong British accent, he greeted me, 'Good morning, Dr Pandit. I am John Houghton, the CEO.'

'Hello, Mr Houghton,' I responded.

I was introduced to the other people in the room, which included a lady officer, Zhang Yifei, and Mr Kris Han, who was the legal head at Mobitrax. I felt a sense of intrigue.

When I was seated, Officer Chen Lun spoke. 'We would like you to meet an employee of this company who is a bit troubled. We want you to speak to her and assess her condition.'

Coming from a police officer, this was a strange request.

*Why were the police interested in an employee issue?* I wondered.

'And why do you think this person is troubled?' I asked, choosing to use the same description.

The officer explained, 'There are still a number of loose ends; until they are tied together, I would not be able to answer your questions with any degree of certainty.'

*Very noncommittal*, I thought.

'Can you tell me something more about this person?' I asked, wanting some background before I met her.

Officer Chen Lun turned towards John, who took the cue and spoke.

'Yang Mi is our IT manager. Her records are decent. I understand she can be very pushy when it comes to going after targets which is good. However, lately, she has been known to be very irritable. HR has also told me that she has been bad-mouthing me in various forums. That's about it.'

'And why was she doing that?' I enquired.

He recollected, 'Well, from what I have heard, it had something to do with me being a foreigner directing the local employees.'

'And are you affected by what she has been saying about you?' I asked, wanting to understand their equations a little better.

He shrugged his shoulders and asserted, 'Of course, not Dr Pandit. I have seen too many like her in my career to be affected by them.'

His body language suggested that he did not really mean what he was saying.

I looked around the room and enquired, 'Anything more I need to know before I meet Yang Mi?'

Everyone looked at each other but remained silent.

Officer Chen Lun spoke. 'Nothing more to add, Dr Pandit. I will request Officer Zhang Yifei to take you to the other room.'

I followed the officer as she led me to an adjacent room. I beckoned her to wait outside and entered the room.

The place seemed like a typical conference room, with a large table and many chairs around it. An overhead projector and a screen suggested that it was a place where meetings would be held. Seated on one of the chairs on the other side of the table was Yang Mi.

She stood up when I entered. A thin woman, probably in her thirties, she had long hair. Dressed in business formals, she looked smart. Her face though was shrouded with fear, and she appeared a bit shaken up.

'Hello, Yang Mi,' I addressed her softly. 'My name is Dr Pandit. I am a psychologist.'

'Hello, Doctor,' she said, and her voice came out in a whisper.

'How are you doing?' I asked gently.

'Why are you asking me?' she questioned me curtly.

I purposely sat down next to her, and said, 'Yang Mi, how are feeling?'

'Feeling!' she exclaimed loudly. 'How would someone feel in a company where no one cares for you.'

A little surprised by the outburst, I asked calmly. 'What makes you say that Yang Mi?'

'The company has been making my life miserable,' she screeched. 'I am required to work twelve hours every day, and even then, the work does not stop. And after all this effort, I am paid a pittance. Don't we have a life outside work? And then we have to take orders from a foreigner. How dare he come into my country and tell me how to work?'

I remained unfazed. 'Yang Mi, you have to calm down,' I said. 'Shouting will not help. You need to tell me clearly.'

She was shaking her head and breathing heavily with all the anger she was spewing out, but she remained silent.

I waited for a while and then interrupted the silence. 'Yang Mi, you have to speak to me. The number of police personnel in the office may be pointing to something serious. And if there is some connection with you, talking to me may be the only way out.'

There was no reaction, but she seemed to be in deep thought, and very soon, a different emotion surfaced. The tears started flowing out in torrents, accompanied with loud wails.

'Please save me, Doctor,' she pleaded in between her tears. 'I don't know what's happening. Please take me away from here.'

'Yang Mi, you have to tell me what happened first,' I persisted. 'That is the only way I can help you.'

'I want to visit the toilet,' she said suddenly and rose from her chair.

'Yang Mi, please wait while I check with the police officer,' I said and stepped out to check with the officer.

Officer Zhang Yifei nodded her agreement when I took her permission and added 'I will accompany you.'

She accompanied the two of us to the washroom. Since Yang Mi was carrying her purse, I suggested. 'Let me hold the purse for you.'

I extended my hand, but Yang Mi held the purse close to her chest and stepped into the washroom. The officer kept her hand on the door to prevent Yang Mi from locking it. From where I was standing, I could see her reflection in the mirror. She seemed to be fidgeting with her purse until she seemed to find what she wanted. She stood still in front of the mirror, holding something in her hand. Suddenly, an alarm bell rang inside my head, and on instinct, I stepped inside the washroom and grabbed her hand. She seemed to be surprised by my sudden intervention and remained motionless. In her hand was a small vial. Before Yang Mi could react, I took it from her hand.

'What are you doing?' Yang Mi screamed loudly.

Showing the vial, I asked, 'What is this, Yang Mi?'

She seemed to search for an answer. 'It's … it's … a … a …'

The door opened, and Officer Zhang Yifei stormed in.

'What's happening?' she asked authoritatively.

'She was having this in her hand,' I said and handed the vial to her.

The officer opened the vial and smelt the contents. Her expression suggested something was amiss.

'Can we move out of this place?' she asked the two of us.

Yang Mi was crying uncontrollably now. I requested the officer to bring her back to the room we were sitting in. She relented and assured me that she would be waiting outside in case I needed her.

'What is happening here?' I wondered. 'Maybe Yang Mi will have some answers.'

I came close to her and said in a stern voice, 'Do you know what you were trying to do? Isn't it so easy to just end your life and get away from your troubles? Did you ever think about your family? Wouldn't they be ashamed and embarrassed when they hear about your cowardly act?'

Yang Mi was now covering her face with her hands as the tears continued to flow. I could sense that these were tears of regret.

'Please, help me,' she pleaded again.

'Tell me what is going on,' I replied sternly, and I looked into her eyes.

'I have committed a mistake,' she finally said. 'A big mistake …'

For the next twenty minutes, she spoke about her financial issues, the system error which she noticed, and her decision to steal the mobile phones. She described how she managed to take the phones out and then sold them to a lady for a good price.'

As she articulated every detail, I could help but admire the audacity of her actions. Although the trigger seemed to be her mother's illness and the escalating cost of treatment, the very fact that she could even think of such a plan seemed unbelievable.

When she had spoken, there was silence. She was waiting for my response, and I, in turn, was too stunned to speak.

'Can you help me?' she pleaded. 'For the sake of my children, please help me.'

'What do you want me to do?' I asked, still figuring out all that I had heard.

'Probably, you can declare that I am insane,' she suggested.

That was a cheeky suggestion, but it made me think. The emotional side of me was suggesting that I accept her request, but my moral side was telling me to stand by the ethics of my profession.

It was no surprise that my moral side won the argument.

'Yang Mi,' I explained, 'I can do no such thing. If you have committed a crime, you have to accept it and face the punishment.'

'You are like the others,' she screamed without any semblance of control on herself. 'Go ahead and put me in jail. That's what all of you want.'

Hearing the screams, Officer Zhang Yifei rushed in and enquired, 'Any problem?'

I replied, 'No, Officer, but I am finished here.'

I turned to Yang Mi and again held her hand. 'Yang Mi, you are a nice person. If you have committed a crime—and the police will determine that—you have to accept it and face the punishment. If not, then justice will be done, and you will be free. I can help you face this situation that you have created for yourself. Probably, we will meet again. Let me just leave you with a thought. This life is a gift from the universe, and we have no right to end it until the universe itself decides that our time is up. Make the most of this gift.'

Yang Mi stared at me as I spoke but remained motionless as I left the room.

As I walked to the CEO's office, I reconsidered my decision. Again, it was my values which came up tops.

'Officer Chen Lun, Mr John Houghton and Mr Kris Han,' I addressed them in the CEO's office. 'I spent some time with Yang Mi, and I feel she is emotionally influenced by the current situation. I could discern a sense of anger, despair, and regret from her continued outburst. From what you have described about her and the few words that she spoke, though, I have no reason to believe that she has a mental condition. However, if she is not handled well, there is a likelihood that she may slip into one.'

The gentlemen and the lady looked at each other.

'Would you need me for anything else?' I asked.

'Thank you so much, Dr Pandit, for coming here at such short notice,' Officer Chen Lun said while extending his hand. 'We will keep you informed.'

I shook his hand and that of the other two gentlemen and the lady officer before leaving the premises.

As I was heading home in the cab, I continued to think about Yang Mi.

I wondered, 'Can circumstances lead a reasonably educated professional woman to an act of stealing? Was she a kleptomaniac? In that case, she may have committed this act earlier as well. There seems to be no mention of that. And the suicide attempt—was she prepared for such an eventuality? If that was the case, then Yang Mi was definitely well in control of herself.'

This was intriguing.

As I reached my destination, I sighed and thought, *Well, I wanted to help her, but I could only do what I was asked to do. Hope she gets justice in more ways than one.*

# 7

The case of Yang Mi was national news. After all, Mobitrax was a big brand in this part of the world. From the day she was arrested, the media covered every aspect of the case. The police charged her for the theft of a large number of mobile phones and for bringing the company into disrepute. The case went into a trial after a few weeks. She was convicted and sentenced to fifteen years in prison.

Details of Yang Mi's personal life, her two children, husband, and ailing mother were splashed on newspapers and local news channels for many days. I could not but pity this lady, who seemed to have a decent corporate career but who, for some reason, had committed a crime and was now facing a long sentence. Something inside me kept telling me that she needed help, and as if on cue, I received a call from the Changi Prison Complex.

'Dr Pandit,' the person said, 'I am Dr Fandi Ahmad, the medical officer at Changi Prison. We understand that you have briefly met Yang Mi before. I would request you to come and meet her again.'

'How is she, Officer?' I asked, pleasantly surprised by this quirk of fate.

'Well, she has been uncontrollable during the past few days, and we feel that these are panic attacks. While we are administering treatment, we feel she also needs the help of a mental-health professional. Her records suggested that you had met her before her conviction, and hence I am calling you.'

I seized the opportunity that probably came my way due to the strong desire of helping Yang Mi.

I reached the biggest prison complex in Singapore early in the morning. After passing through the necessary security procedures, I was escorted to the medical centre, where I met Dr Fandi Ahmad. He briefed me about her frequent panic attacks and led me to the doctor's visiting room. He asked me to wait there while he would arrange for Yang Mi to be brought to the centre.

When Yang Mi entered the room, she was so unlike the person that I had met a few weeks before. The lady in front of me was frail, her face had shrunk, with the cheekbones clearly visible. There were dark circles around her eyes, and her eyelids were puffy. Her shoulders were drooping, and her hands seemed so much thinner. Clearly, the past few weeks had taken a toll on her health.

'Hello, Yang Mi,' I greeted her. 'Do you remember me?'

She stared at me blankly, as her mind may have been sifting through the many faces she had seen over the past few weeks during the trial.

'I am Dr Pandit,' I said. 'We met at the Mobitrax office.'

A slight change in her expression hinted at recognition, but it stopped there. She turned her gaze to the floor and remained motionless.

It felt strange that here I was thinking about this person almost every day, and this other person hardly seemed to recognise me.

'A lot has happened since we last met, Yang Mi,' I said softly. 'Nothing can be done about it. You can, however, change the course of events in your future, but only if you want to.'

She looked up at me, and I could catch a faint smile escape her lips.

I continued in a soft tone, 'I am a therapist who helps people discover themselves, and in the past thirty years, I have helped many people who were in worse situations come out of their misery and lead a normal life. Don't you want to lead a normal life again? Don't you want to spend time with your daughters? Don't you want to be with your sick mother? Don't you want to hold your husband's hands and grow old with him?' The tone of my voice increased with every question, as they intended to pierce her staid exterior and bring forth some of her raw emotions.

The soliloquy seemed to have made an impact as her expressions began to change. Slowly the tears made an appearance and very soon they turned into a flood.

I was relieved in a way since I could now address the emotional part of her.

I continued, 'The world may be saying many things about you, but I want you to tell me what you are going through.'

She was crying her heart out.

I went and sat next to her in an attempt to comfort her. She suddenly turned and hugged me tightly while continuing to cry loudly. I put my arms around her and stroked her head gently.

After, what seemed like an eternity, she stepped back from the embrace. The tears had stopped, and she seemed to have let out her pent-up emotions.

And then there was an outburst.

'I don't want to live,' she screamed. 'My daughters must be ashamed of me. My mother is dying, and I can't be with her. I am of no use to anyone lying in this prison. I would rather die and free everyone from the pain I have caused them.'

A while after I waked in, I spoke.

'Yang Mi, you had a good life. You had a nice family—a supportive husband and lovely children. You had a nice job as well. What happened thereafter was a result of your bad choices. If your bad choices could lead you to this place, some good choices can also take you out of here. And taking your life is definitely not one of them.'

She was listening.

'Tell me what you are feeling. Let the guilt, the remorse, the regret all come out today,' I urged.

She remained silent.

'What do you have to lose?' I implored. 'You will be locked up in this prison for fifteen years. Do you even know how long that is? If you sit here and do nothing about it, you will not be able to see your daughters grow up. The only option available for you Yang Mi is to talk and share your innermost feelings. I may be your last hope. And if you don't talk, even I will be gone.'

The continued barrage of words worked. Finally, she spoke. And when she did, she poured her heart out.

She described her childhood, her teenage years, her marriage, the birth of her two girls, her career, and her passions. She described her love for travel, shopping, eating in fancy restaurants, and living the good life.

'When my mother was diagnosed with cancer, I felt like the end of the world,' she confessed. 'I loved my mother and wanted to give her the best treatment, but I also could see my dreams being shattered. I felt very guilty about these thoughts. How could I even think about my dreams when my mother was suffering? And that is when an opportunity presented itself. I felt it was God's way of telling me to go ahead with it. For the company, the loss of a few mobile phones did not mean anything, whereas for me, it was a lifeline. I was scared initially. I was very scared. I would also feel bad that I was stealing, but slowly, I realised how easy it was. I was making decent money from it. I was now able to take care of my mother's treatment and even save some money. I felt that life was so much better now.'

Yang Mi was reminiscing her past and she poured out every detail.

'Didn't you ever feel scared that you will get caught?' I asked her.

'Very scared,' she admitted, 'but I needed the money, and I was ready to take the risk. I could not sleep at night thinking of the consequences. I know the penalty for such a crime, but I was more worried about the shame that my family would undergo. And there was only one way out.'

She paused and I asked, 'And what was that?'

'I ... I ... decided to keep a vial of cyanide in my purse,' she confessed. 'I decided to consume it whenever I get caught.'

'That was extreme,' I though. I now had an explanation for the episode in the company toilet.

'Wasn't there a sense of regret?' I asked.

'Many times. And I tried to stop,' she admitted. 'But I could not. So, I called the HR manager anonymously and told her about someone stealing the mobile phones.'

'You called the HR manager?' I asked, surprised by this admission.

She nodded.

'And what happened?' I probed.

'Nothing, absolutely nothing,' she snapped. 'One would have thought that a big company like Mobitrax would tighten their processes, but no one was bothered.'

'Why did you call the HR head?' I enquired, still unsure of this action. 'Wouldn't that have made it difficult for you to take any more mobile phones from the warehouse?'

'Yes ... precisely,' she said. 'Then I would not have to convince myself to stop, but that did not happen. So I called the warehouse manager.'

'And?' I asked, becoming more and more intrigued with her strange sequence of actions.

'And he did nothing as well,' she said sarcastically. 'In this global public listed company, no one cares about anything else but their targets. If that is achieved, nothing else matters. I slog days and nights, but what has the company given me in return?'

She was all worked up and spewed venom with every word she spoke.

'And then I called the CEO,' she confessed.

I couldn't believe what I was hearing. Here was someone who had committed a crime and was calling the very people from whom she had stolen to tell them about the crime.

'I hate him' she declared, even as I tried to figure out the new detail that was coming to light, 'but I hoped that at least he would do something to tighten up the process.'

'Yang Mi,' I asked, 'all these people you called would have taken some actions which would have prevented you from stealing the phones. But did you not think that they would also report you to the police?'

'How would they recognise me?' she questioned me and said, 'I would always call from a public telephone and even use a handkerchief to disguise my voice.'

*She was not that smart after all*, I thought.

I started to explain that she was being naive but stopped. I had no intention to prove her naivety; rather, I wanted her to move forward with her life.

'Yang Mi, listen to me carefully,' I explained. 'I believe that the company was putting a lot of pressure on you. You were slogging every day of the week, and you were unhappy with your compensation. Let's assume that all of this is true. What were the choices available with you at that point? You took one of those choices and ended up here. What were the other choices?'

She gazed at the floor and seemed deep in thought. After some moments of silence, she spoke.

'I could have quit,' she thought aloud.

'Probably, or probably not,' I clarified. 'That was a choice but then you had a family and your mother's medical expenses. So, quitting may not have been a good option. How about searching for another job?'

'Ah,' Yang Mi uttered, trying to understand what I was saying.

'Probably that was also not practical, because you hardly had any time from your daily chores,' I concluded. 'What I am trying to explain is that at every point of time, you have more than one choice. The course of your life is determined by the choices you make. If you had spent some time considering all the choices you had and looked at the pros and cons of each, there is a possibility you may have chosen a different path.'

She was listening intently.

'While the stress at work may have been the trigger for whatever happened, there is only one person responsible for where you are today,' I explained, 'and that is you. The earlier you accept it, the faster will be the journey to your new life.'

Yang Mi put her head in her cupped hands and remained silent.

There was a knock on the door to the room. I checked my watch and realised that I had been there for more than ninety minutes.

Dr Fandi Ahmad opened the door and peeped in.

'Can I come in?' he asked.

'Of course, Doctor,' I replied. 'We were finishing anyway.'

I looked at Yang Mi and said, 'Yang Mi, you are a good person and deserve a good life. As we discussed just now, you have many choices—even at this point in time. Think of them and choose the one which will help you achieve your dreams.'

I bid goodbye to Yang Mi and to the doctor. On the way back home, I recalled the conversation.

'Did she actually make those phone calls? I did not recall reading about the calls in the many news reports published in the print media. I decided to find out. I called the board number of Mobitrax and asked to be connected to the HR manager.

With the initial introductions done, I went straight to the subject.

'Miss Chin,' I said, 'your ex-employee Yang Mi is in prison for a crime which she has confessed to. Her state of mind during the last few weeks has been extremely fragile, and there is a danger that she may slip into a mental condition. As a therapist, I feel that she needs help. I have spent some time with her in the prison and heard her side of the story. I would like to hear the company's side to determine the further course of action.'

Miss Chin thought about the request and replied, 'Dr Pandit, I appreciate the work you are doing. However, I am bound by company policies and cannot divulge details of our employees.'

That was not an unexpected response and I was prepared for it.

'I completely understand your position, Miss Chin,' I acknowledged. 'I will provide a recommendation from the prison medical staff. I suppose that will help.'

'Yes, Doctor,' she replied and her voice revealed her eagerness to help.

We decided on a mutually convenient date and time.

## 8

Miss Felicia Chin seemed very young for her role as an HR manager. She seemed like one of the smart professionals who graduate from management schools and climb a curated path up the corporate ladder. She seemed very warm, and everything about her conveyed an intent to help, which was in line with my perception after our call a couple of days earlier.

'Miss Chin,' I asked after the initial icebreakers, 'what can you tell me about Yang Mi?'

'As per the HR records, she has been a decent performer. While she has not always met her performance targets, she has not been too far away either. Over the years, there have been a few complaints against her. Other employees have reported that she can be too pushy, she loses her temper very often, and sometimes she even talks ill about the company. None of these complaints were considered serious enough for HR to issue an official warning letter. However, on our request, her managers have discussed these complaints with her at various times.'

'Would you be aware of any particular employee who was at the receiving end of Yang Mi's outbursts?' I probed.

'All the complaints were raised by different employees,' she responded and clarified, 'if that's what you wanted to know.'

I acknowledged her efforts.

'Thanks for the details,' I said and asked the question which was constantly rearing in my head. 'Let me ask you one last question. I was told that Yang Mi called you one afternoon and informed you about the mobile phones being stolen from the company premises. Is that true?'

'Yes,' she replied with a smile, 'I did receive a call from an unknown number, and the person did not reveal her identity.'

*Oh!* I thought. *She was speaking the truth.*

'And did you do anything about it?' I asked.

'Well, I had briefly mentioned it to my manager, but he did not feel that it warranted any serious thought. We believe that our processes are pretty tight, and any discrepancy of this magnitude would have been identified,' she confessed.

It was my turn to respond with a smile.

'And apparently, they were not,' I said.

She nodded her head sheepishly.

'And I presume the other call that she made to your warehouse manager was also brushed aside,' I enquired.

'I guess so,' she said. 'Mr Irfan Mohammed would have also thought along the same lines.'

I sat back on my chair.

'Miss Chin,' I asked, 'what lessons have we learnt from this case?'

She pondered the question in earnest and responded, 'Dr Pandit, the case has broken the myth that our processes are watertight and there is nothing to improve. Let me admit that in the quest for achieving our numbers, we seem to be compromising with our policies and standards. The biggest lesson for me as an HR manager is to be more in touch with my people. In the quest for meeting their targets, every employee is under stress, which may lead them into actions which may not be in line with our values. In hindsight, if we could have facilitated the process by which someone like Yang Mi could have channelised her stress, the outcomes could have been different.'

I was impressed with her reading of the situation and the inferences drawn. The last part of what she said was what I was looking for. As a mental health professional, I can see the impact of workplace pressures on the human mind. It is high time that the corporates identify this as their topmost priority when framing their policies.

I appreciated Miss Felicia Chin for her support and wished her the very best for her career ahead.

My next port of call was the CEO, Mr John Houghton.

Mr Houghton seemed the stereotypical Englishman, well groomed, articulate, very expressive with his gestures but very measured with his words.

'It was not a very pleasant call,' he admitted with a smirk when I asked him to share his thoughts when he received a call from Yang Mi.

'Did you feel at that time that her revelation had some merit?' I enquired.

'Not at all,' he stated. 'I was more concerned with the nature of the call and that too at the odd hour.'

'Are there any lessons to be learnt from this case?' I probed.

'Not really.' He frowned. 'Do you think her actions would not have been identified otherwise?'

'Would they have?' I countered.

'You would be mistaken if you think that her actions have contributed to any process improvements,' he declared with an air of confidence. 'We believe in continuous process improvements and any lacunae if at all they exist would come to light very soon.'

I posed a few more questions, but the man seemed adept at brushing them aside.

While the HR manager had admitted to their failings, it seemed so unlike the leader of the company to also not do the same.

During that week, I visited Yang Mi's home, where I met her husband, Deng Xiao, and her ailing mother. Her daughters, aged 4 and 8, were too young to understand the details, but they seemed to miss their mother so much.

Deng Xiao seemed morose and struggling to cope with the avalanche that had hit their small, happy family.

He shared his feelings in an emotional conversation.

'Yang Mi was a wonderful wife and mother. She was very ambitious and probably that was her undoing. She wanted everything fast. She would be unhappy when her friends travelled abroad and would keep dreaming about travelling around the world one day. I would tell her to be happy with what we have. We have lovely kids, a decent house, and good jobs, but she always wanted more.'

'Did you ever suspect that she was taking away the mobile phones from the company?' I asked.

'Not at all,' he confessed. 'She would leave for work early in the morning, and I presumed it is the work pressure. I never realised that she was visiting some shops that sold the phones. Why did she have to do that? Sometimes, I admonish myself for not being around to support her.'

He broke down, and I felt sorry for him and the children.

I resolved to do something more for Yang Mi, and it did not take long for another opportunity to present itself.

## 9

I was called to the Changi Prison Complex again.

Yang Mi had had another a panic attack, and this time, it was more severe than the many times it had occurred earlier. I brought my good friend and wonderful psychiatrist Dr Betty Chang with me. I had taken special permission from the prison authorities to have a series of sessions with Yang Mi. Over the next few weeks, Dr Betty and I worked with Yang Mi to bring her mind to a state of acceptance of her current situation. It did not help that apart from the sessions, there was very little support available to complement the mind shift achieved during the sessions.

During my discussions with Dr Fandi Ahmad, I realised that the prison had weekly activities, such as yoga, pottery, and other crafts. I was told that most of the inmates avoided these activities and would rather be left alone. I suggested some ideas to make these activities more interesting. I also impressed upon Dr Fandi Ahmad and his team, the need to ensure that Yang Mi participated in these activities regularly.

Slowly but surely, with a combination of therapy, some counselling, some talking, a lot of listening and her participation in other activities, she started coming around. Within six months, she was more receptive to the therapy sessions. She would express herself more freely. She would share her experiences while doing various activities and her feelings when her family would visit her. She was more cooperative in prison, and the frequency of her panic attacks significantly reduced. But she insisted that I continue to visit her. We would talk about many things, my cases, and her job, and we would share a laugh.

'How could you even think of calling up your CEO?' I asked one day.

'That should be logged in the *Guinness Book of World Records* as a new form of suicide,' she declared, and we had a hearty laugh.

Once she started opening up and expressing herself more, her health also started improving.

The big news came around a year into her sentence when an excited Dr Fandi Ahmad called me one day.

'Dr Pandit,' he exclaimed, 'there is some good news for you.'

'I am waiting, Doctor,' I said in anticipation. 'Go on.'

'Yang Mi's sentence has been reduced to eight years due to her good behaviour,' he shared. 'Since she has already served more than a year, she now has less than seven years remaining. And you deserve the credit for it.'

'That's wonderful news, Doctor!' I exclaimed. 'Yes, I have worked with her and helped her turn around, but you and the other jail officials need to be appreciated as well. I will personally come over and do that.'

I visited the prison a few days later, and as soon as the warden brought her to the room, Yang Mi came and hugged me tightly. She started sobbing uncontrollably and kept mumbling in between her tears.

When she was through with her words and the tears, I said to her, 'Thank you for everything you said, but I couldn't understand a word of it.'

We couldn't control our laughter, and for that brief moment, we could have been two friends having a good time in a park.

With gratitude clearly visible in her eyes, Yang Mi said, 'Dr Pandit, I cannot thank you enough. If it were not for you, I might not be alive today. From the day I met you, my days in the prison cell seemed so different. I now look forward to the next day, since it will be another day closer to my release. And now that day is even closer. To be precise, it is only 6 years and 326 days away. That's not too far away, is it?'

'No, it is not, my dear,' I replied, 'It is so much better than 13 years and 326 days.'

I continued to visit her regularly. More than therapy, we would just have conversations. I would also visit her family from time to time. During this period, cancer got the better of her mother, and Yang Mi was given a few hours of parole to spend a few moments with her mother's mortal remains.

As she hugged her daughters and said her goodbyes, she had one last word for me.

She said with a smile, 'I am looking forward to the day I will be released. You have given me a reason to live.'

## 10

Yang Mi could have been any normal working woman, who had dreams when they are young, but the pressure of work, married life, children, and possibly old parents to care for pushed these dreams to some corner of her mind from where they could never be retrieved. Some manage to do it in this life, some succumb to the pressures and a majority just go through life, bereft of any desires.

Most of my clients have been victims of the environment that they were a part of, and some were born with traits which did not allow them to define their own existence. Yang Mi, on the other hand, was a victim of her own wrong choices. At every point in our lives, we make choices. If they are informed choices, there is a high probability of them turning out to be right, but there is no certainty. The turning point in Yang Mi's life was the choice she made when she became aware of the programming error. From that point onwards, every choice she made compounded the problem and her subsequent choices were all leading to only one outcome. In the heavy glare of an obsession for a good life, she could not see this outcome, and she continued to tread on a path of no return.

In her pursuit of good life, every person who got in the way was deemed a villain. If a team member was not working hard enough, she considered that as harming her goal achievement, and hence her bonus. That made her lose her temper. It did not take too long for her to believe that the entire company was against her and her dreams. While her conscience pricked her from time to time during the initial days, the presence of a villain—the company, in this case—made it easy for her subconscious mind to justify her actions. From there on in, every event which did not happen in her favour was the villain's doing. Through this shift of responsibility, she was giving away control of her mind and its ability to make further choices.

However, there is another point of view which needs to be considered.

She had been a loyal employee of the company, and as a manager, she would be privy to the internal working of the company. Even their HR manager admitted that in the quest for achieving targets, the basic values of the company were being compromised. Through her actions, which may seem unethical, was she subconsciously trying to get these wrongs corrected? If that was indeed the case, she had achieved her objective since the company did take measures to review and tighten their processes after Yang Mi's case came to light. What if this realisation had dawned on them a little earlier?

With the growing pressure on a working professional, especially a woman with a family, every corporation would have employees like Yang Mi; it is imperative that there are enough measures to identify them and prevent them from making such wrong choices. A question that every corporation need to ask themselves is 'Are we doing enough to take care of our employees?'

This was a case which was all over the media during the trial and subsequent sentencing. This also became a case study at the Institute of Mental Health.

## PREETI PANDIT'S BLOGS

## 1—FEAR FACTORS

Fear and anxiety are your biggest hurdles to living a happy and balanced life. In this write-up, we take an in-depth look at the factors that cause fear and also at ways to overcome it.

Fear is a mental construct which is based on some past unhappy moments or just pure imagination. Worry is the incubation chamber for fear because worry, if unchecked, will always lead to fear being unleashed. As a result of this mental state, it always causes the person to live on the defensive. Some religions use fear as a tool to instil good values among their followers. Many fears are merely a result of some emotional anguish, and these fears seek to destroy our peace and torment our minds if not checked in time.

*How Does Fear Operate?*

Here is a simple story that can give us an insight into the working of fear. A young man on a scholarship at a top university in New York wanted to complete his course as soon as possible. Often neglecting dinner, he stayed back late to complete assignments. On his way to the hostel, it would be usually cold and dark, and he could hardly find food. Even if he could, he would be too tired to eat. After many weeks of sleeping through hunger, he fell sick and was hospitalised. The fear of darkness, winter, and hunger crept into his system. Now, whenever winter sets in, it triggers a fear with emotional pain and pressure. The bad experience of the winter of hunger has conditioned his system to respond unnaturally.

*Defining Worry*

In mental health circles, worry is often called the common cold of emotions. It is also a part of a much larger emotional challenge. Serious forms are called 'panic anxiety.' This usually starts suddenly and occurs in people who are high achievers, who often place themselves under enormous stress. Worry becomes unhealthy and destructive when it persists for too long or when it never leads to constructive solutions. At some time or other, we all go through periods of worry as life throws surprises and challenges at us. Loss of a beloved one, job stress, and health problems are all threatening to us and cause worry which finally leads to fear. Worry kicks in an important signal, which can be used to take corrective action. So a healthy step is to find out exactly what is happening with your body and begin making plans to overcome its adverse effects before it can rule (and ruin) your life.

*How to Overcome Worry?*

One strategy to overcome worry is through awareness and professional counselling. We learn by observing how our parents and role *models react and respond to life's situations.* One should learn to face challenges and opportunities alike without getting stressed by the outcome. People can recover easily from anxiety and worries if they keep their expectations at a realistic level and also cultivate an attitude of acceptance.

*How Are Fear, Anxiety, and Worry Correlated?*

Anxiety leads to worry, which, in turn, leads to fear. So the key is to manage your anxieties and nip them in the bud. Most people are generally anxious when they are ignorant and are burdened by expectations from family, friends, and society in general. Failure and emotional damage in these pursuits can lead to developing fear.

*How to Overcome Fear?*

It requires a very cool mind and strong determination to overcome fear. First, you have to analyse what you are afraid of. If you are struggling with anxiety attacks, carefully review the sequence of events that preceded the fearful moments. If the same event were to happen again, how would you react? Would you be better off with a different response? Was the fear just a mind construct, or was it real? If it was just a mind construct, throw it away. If it was real, then courage has to be used to overcome it. An intervention by a psychologist can be very helpful in going through this process.

## 2—PARENTING SKILLS

*How Can I Be a Better Parent?*

Parenting process entails the essential task of nurturing self-esteem and confidence in the children. It involves imparting good values and imbibing morality in them. Parents-to-be must have adequate preparedness, resources, and support to guide them through the child-rearing process.

There needs to be a constant flow of new ideas and inputs to match the rapidly changing society, setting new demands on parents. There is a lot of learning to be done in this parenting process. If you are very orderly, children will make you chaotic. Children are best to break your boundaries. Your children teach you a lot that others may not be able to. The first thing for us is to observe a child and his tendencies, and thereafter, it is a two-way journey.

*1. Communicate Clearly with Children*

Children need to learn how to communicate well. You can help them improve their communication skills by encouraging reading as well as talking clearly. Give simple instructions and correct messages. Match the child's language; children's speeches and approaches are developing, so parents need to use language that they will understand. Parents should encourage them to expand what they say. For example, when a two-year-old says, 'Cat on tree,' parents can help by saying, 'Yes, the cat is on the tree, and look: it jumped down.' Give positive messages.

## 2. Allow Children the Space and Opportunity to Find Their Own Individuality

Helping them find their dream and persuading them to walk towards the dream is the biggest challenge for parents. So, expose them to multifarious activities. This is ideally done when a child is at age 10 or 11. You should encourage the child to try activities relating to science, arts, maths, music, and social skills and expose them to all the faculties including doing service. The left brain as well as the right brain must be nourished. The concept of Saraswati, goddess of learning, is amazing. If you look at the symbol of Saraswati, there is a musical instrument, a book and a rosary in her hands. The book symbolises nourishing the left brain, the musical instrument symbolises nourishing the right brain, and rosary symbolises the meditative aspect. So, knowledge, music, and meditation—all three are required to make the education complete. Also, encourage them to ask questions. On one Sunday, give them some chocolates and ask them to distribute to the poorest people. Once or twice in a year, take them to a slum area and ask them to do social service. This will enhance and develop their personality and make them more all-rounded and compassionate.

## 3. Listen Effectively

Listen to what your children are trying to say to you—verbally as well as through other means. They too have their own fears and insecurities and need constant reassurances to build their confidence. What may seem inconsequential or insignificant to you may be a real issue for them as they grapple with it.

## 4. Deal with Misbehaviour Issues

Understand the cause of the children's attention-seeking behaviour. If the behaviour is purely attention-seeking, don't give it undue importance. Ignore it, if possible. Give positive attention and encouragement at other more appropriate times. Set limits, but withdraw from the conflicts. Give a child a sense of power and control in appropriate situations by allowing the child to choose or make decisions.

Make sure that they interact with various age groups, which helps them to avoid misbehaviour. How do they interact with someone of their own age group? Children who have an inferiority complex like to interact more with the younger ones and try to run away from older ones and even try to avoid their equals. People with a superiority complex try to shun younger ones and only want to relate to older ones. They are not good communicators in either case.

## 5. Cultivate Trust

Children have a trusting tendency by nature. But their trust can be easily broken. Check the message your child is trying to convey; you need to look into that. Do they trust themselves? Do they have enough confidence in themselves?

A healthy child will have three kinds of trust: trust in the divinity, trust in the goodness of people, and trust in oneself. A healthy child will not think that everybody is a thief or everybody is bad. He or she won't indulge this sort of paranoia. A healthy child knows that people are good. A healthy child has trust in him or herself and trust in the unseen power of God/Divinity (i.e., some higher power). These three types of trust can make a child confident. These are the ingredients that make a very talented and well-rounded child. To nurture them, we need to bring about these tendencies in them. If you keep telling children that everyone is a cheat, the child loses his trust in the people around and the society in general. Their personality, talents, and communication skills will shrink, and they can never blossom.

## 6. Discourage Sibling Rivalry

As parents, you have a duty to treat all your children equally. Never show even the slightest iota of favouritism. You should do everything you can to convey the message that each child is unique and has his or her own special strengths and talents and that we love each one equally. This will go a great way towards neutralising any sibling rivalry.

## 7. Spend Family Time Together

When you have no control over your own moods, it is difficult to make a mood or create an atmosphere just for the sake of children. But we need to make an effort. Here is an exercise to do every day which can help. When you come back from work, the first thing you do is clap with them, play, or laugh. It may look a little artificial for one or two days. But later on, it will become a breakthrough for you and your children. Sit and have food with the whole family as often as possible, at least three to four times a week. And while having food, don't tell them they are bad. While serving them food, don't put down their moods. There is a time to tell them when they are wrong but never at the dining table. Also, to encourage interaction with other family members, give them some responsibility of youngsters and sometimes some responsibility to do something for older ones, by which you can bridge their generation gap.

## 8. *Play a Balancing Role*

When children are very positive about their friends, give them a little caution but not too much. If they are very negative about some friends, show them that there is something positive also. Participate with them and learn from them. So, you have to have a balancing act whenever a child swings too much to the left or too much to the right. And you can play a very important role here.

## 9. *Enjoy Parenthood*

Parenting can be the most wonderful thing one can do, and successful parenting causes people to grow and change. Parents are tested in many ways that require creative tools or thinking to help in the process. Because everyone is different, what works for one parent may not work for another. As children grow and change, parents need to adopt new methods and approaches, which can work well for the relationship. Children look up to parents for guidance and get their cue for desirable behaviour and values in life.

## 3—MEMORY ENHANCEMENT AND TRAINING

Memory is an important element in our lives. It plays a crucial role in helping us successfully accomplish all our endeavours. In any profession, a well-trained memory can prove to be a priceless asset. With a trained memory, one can approach work with rejuvenated confidence, communicate appropriately, coordinate with others effectively, organise time efficiently, and perform assigned tasks with a clear view of the overall objectives. Learn more about this powerful instrument and how you can make it better.

*Where Is Our Memory Located?*

Memory is located in the hippocampus, a major component of the human brain and also of other mammals. This part of the brain plays an important role in the consolidation of information from short-term memory to long-term memory.

*What Determines a Good or Bad Memory?*

There is no such thing as a *good memory* or a *bad memory*. All human beings are gifted with an equal capacity to memorise things. To start with, everyone has an excellent memory. The distinction between people having 'good' memory and 'bad' memory depends on how well they put their memory to use. (Even the most effective mechanism shall not yield a satisfactory result if it is operated in faulty ways).

Memory is a three-stage process, namely, *registration*, *retention*, and *recall*. These are also known as the three R's of memory. Registration is the most crucial stage which decides whether the information can be retained and recalled. Most memory problems are a direct result of improper registration. Retention is the ability to recognise what has been learnt or experienced. Recall is to summon back the subject or situation at hand.

*It is commonly believed that if you do not revise the information which you learn, you lose a great deal of it with the passage of time.*

Memory is of two kinds—short-term memory (STM) and long-term memory (LTM). Whatever new information you learn enters the brain via short-term memory. If there is no deliberate effort to transfer the information from STM to LTM, the information fades out from STM.

To avoid this, one needs to revise the information a second time to ensure that vital information is converted into LTM.

The process of forgetting starts soon after the first-time input of information, and a vast majority of whatever is learnt is forgotten within twenty-four hours of learning. For longer-term retention, a person should do the following:

1. First round of revision after ten minutes of learning
2. Second round of revision within twenty-four hours of learning
3. Third revision within a week of learning
4. Fourth revision within a month of learning
5. Fifth revision within two months of learning

*What Techniques Facilitate Retention and Developing an LTM?*

Use of written words, such as maintaining a diary for important information like names of clients, customers, appointments, meetings, business schedules, telephone numbers, statistical data and dates, is very useful.

Using the 'association method' to memorise information is also helpful. Relating new information to existing memorised reference points leads to easy retention. It lends meaning to the new matter, classifying newly learnt information, and categorising them into words related to existing information.

Focus on retaining important information that is useful for work, family, and daily routine. In your free time, communicate effectively with the brain by recalling the important events and information. Avoid forgetfulness by scanning the recordings in the diary at the end of each day and also once a week; finally, review it once a month. Keep track of the heaps of information and comprehend more effectively whatever is read. This exercise of recording and recalling will lead to a stronger memory. Many fancy instruments are available in this century to write and record important data, such as smartphones, USB drives, and laptops.

*Does the Use of Pictures Help in Creating Better LTM?*

The brain remembers pictures better than words. That is the reason advertisers use more pictures to create their marketing campaigns. For a person, it is easy to recall information which is associated with pictures. Messages given as digital movies using action with pictures accelerate the memorisation process. It is futile to try speeding up the learning process by simply spending longer hours at a stretch, as many do when they're anxious. The human brain cannot effectively concentrate continuously on the influx of information.

The longer the time spent on learning without a break, the greater the chances of forgetting. The remedy to this problem is to break the learning time into units of thirty minutes each, by introducing breaks of two to five minutes. This intermission accelerates learning, which helps the brain to organise the material taken in thirty minutes earlier. During the break, one can either relax or unconsciously revise what was learnt before the break.

## 4—UNDERSTANDING ADDICTION

*What Causes Addiction and How Can We Help It?*

Addiction is a complex illness that involves biochemical processes in the brain, especially in the midbrain and parts of the prefrontal cortex. Like other chronic illnesses, this one too, if detected and treated in its early stages, bears favourable results and avoids further complications. A range of treatments are available that are both accessible and quite affordable. Involvement of the patient's family and close friends in his or her treatment and recovery has proved very useful. Here are a few common types of addiction.

*Types of Addictions*

1. *Substance addiction* leads to dependence and regular use of products like heroin, alcohol, nicotine, and synthetic drugs. The individual's attraction to and need for these substances grow over time, making it difficult for the person to live a normal and healthy life.

2. *Process or behavioural addiction*, such as excessive gambling, multiple sex relationships, having and displaying a particular type of emotions repeatedly, as well as excessive eating and work habits, are some addictions in this category. Such addictions pull a person away from his or her normal behaviour. It is also found that an addiction such as gambling is an illness which can never really be cured but only contained or transformed. Under gambling alone, there are different types of addicts who act differently. The antisocial gambler pursues a motive by the act of cheating. He or she enjoys doing this and uses it for relaxation and recreation. Another type is the social gambler who plays for social recognition. According to this gambler, the more he or she achieves through gambling, the better he or she is positioned among peers. A more severe addiction is seen in problem gambling, which is a persistent and recurrent maladaptive behaviour that disrupts personal, family, or vocational well-being.

3. *Game addiction* is regarded as a psychological addiction from the overuse of video games, such that the addict exhibits certain symptoms common to addiction, as well as neglecting his or her real life for the online life. Symptoms of people suffering from game addiction include a sense of euphoria while playing cyber games; inability to stop computer activity; craving more time on

the computer; feelings of depression; neglect of family, friends, and social activities; lying; and using it to escape from problems.

## How Does a Person Become an Addict?

There are many factors involved with such behaviour. This can happen because of cognition—irrational thinking, peer pressure, family abuse, unitary family systems, growing up in an extremely critical environment, and facing constant rejection or emotionally unavailable parents. Families that overemphasise status, overvalue money, or create an extremely competitive environment at home may lead someone towards addictive behaviour. Exposure to gambling and alcohol at an early age also increases these chances. The situation worsens if the parents are habituated as well.

Misaligned habits and poor coping strategies in life lead to imbalances of chemicals in the body. Once an addict drops the addiction activity or action, it causes irritation in the body, as the person is unable to manage his or her mental balance. In due course, this may even damage the brain.

## Why Is It Difficult to Get Rid of Addiction?

With their current anxiety levels, people always look for ways to escape the mental disturbance, even if they are dysfunctional options. And once they find the escape route through these methods, they latch on to it and are reluctant to give them up easily. To them, it's the easiest way out.

Some of the obstacles to positive change are the inability to cope up with shame or guilt, loneliness, depression, fear, anxiety, and the sheer uncertainty associated with such a state. Other obstacles are lack of confidence in the self to make such a transition. Further, a lack of understanding (vision) of what is needed and the inability to see personal or professional benefits of the change also act as obstacles. In fact, some common questions trouble them: Do I have the strength to come out of this addiction? What's wrong with the way things are?

## How Can Addicts Mend Their Ways?

Each person possesses an innate powerful potential for change, and a therapist can inspire this change. Motivation is defined as the probability that a person will initiate, continue, and adhere to a specific behaviour. There are four basic principles of motivational therapy.

1. *Express empathy*. Accept the *person* but not the *behaviour*. Show that you understand what drove the person into substance use while identifying the various feelings and human yearnings behind such behavioural patterns.

2. *Develop discrepancy*. Create and amplify, in the client's mind, a discrepancy between the present behaviour and broader goals. Encourage the client to express negative feelings about gambling. Tell them about the downside of such addictions. Help them to perceive discrepancy at different levels. For example, if they continue this addiction as before, how do they see themselves years from now? What sorts of things are important? How does gambling fit in with their goals (positive self)?

3. *Avoid argument*. Arguments are counterproductive. They only force people to defend the behaviour that they are trying to change. Set up being on *their* side. Resistance is a signal to change the strategies.

4. *Support self-efficacy*. By eliciting and supporting hope and optimism, try to bring attention to the client's assets and strengths; acknowledge progress, no matter how small it is. Set targets which are easily achievable. Try to offer a range of alternatives.

*What Are the Various Techniques Used by a Therapist?*

A therapist's optimism can powerfully influence a client's motivation and outcome.

*Behaviour therapy* is very commonly used by therapists to cure addictions. It is based on experimentally derived principles of learning, which are systematically applied to help people change their maladaptive behaviours. It deals with clients' current problems and factors influencing them, as opposed to an analysis of possible historical factors (past).

Behaviour therapy also emphasises the self-control approach in which clients learn self-management strategies. Therapists frequently train clients to initiate, conduct, and evaluate their own therapy.

Therapists strive to develop culture-specific procedures and obtain their clients' adherence and cooperation. They enhance self-management skills with the expectation that their clients will be responsible for transferring what they learn in the therapist's office to their everyday lives.

Governments across the nations are constantly coming up with new programs and setting aside money for addiction research as well as funding public educational talks and assessment and treatment of addictive disorders by a multidisciplinary team of psychiatrists, counsellors, and social workers.

## 5—HEALING THROUGH BOOKS

When people are affected by trauma or disaster, they may find it difficult to express their thoughts and feelings in words. An intervention by a psychotherapist may be helpful but suffers from limitations of time and costs. However, a good psychotherapist can recommend relevant books to fill in the gaps and develop a self-help routine for the affected person. Such books can be stories about people who suffered similar trauma and disasters and how they successfully tackled them. Alternatively, books on meditation and spirituality can be recommended to help address inner conflict. The psychotherapist has to be extremely well read and should know how to use book therapy in his or her advice and counselling.

*How Do Counsellors Use Books as Therapeutic Tools?*

Book psychotherapy uses stories and drawings to process difficult emotions. Stories and symbolic images can help people connect to their deeper feelings that they find difficult to talk about. The combination of face-to-face counselling and book psychotherapy can help patients move past emotional issues that keep them stuck. We are all familiar with the story of Helen Keller—a deaf and blind person in the 1880s who went on to attain celebrity status. We have the story of Oprah Winfrey, who was physically abused in her early life but is now a big celebrity in the USA. We have the story of Steve Jobs, who never had an easy life yet achieved the pinnacle of success. The job of a psychotherapist is to inspire positivity in the mindsets of affected people and help them live better lives.

*How Does Meditation with Book Psychotherapy Help Patients?*

Meditative practice enables a patient to relax and draw on positive energy, and it encourages them to draw on their inner resources. Those who experience trauma often suffer from depression or anxiety, and the result can be a long period of low energy and enthusiasm. When the body is relaxed through meditation, positive thoughts and actions can result and lead to positive change. Meditative practice when combined with creative experience, such as book psychotherapy, can enable patients to process their emotions and begin to enjoy life. Book psychotherapy, under proper guidance from a psychotherapist, provides the opportunity to speed up healing, transformation, and personal growth. The use of therapeutic intervention by asking patients to explore drawings, paintings, and expressive messages as symbolic language and then analysing them for treating deeper emotional and inner conflicts can go a long way in instilling the right mindset in people afflicted with negativity and depression. Images enhance the verbal exchange between the patient and therapist and assist people in emotional distress to achieve insights, resolve inner conflicts, enhance coping, and formulate new perceptions about the problem. Thereafter, the tool of book psychotherapy can be used deftly in between counselling to reduce stress.

*A Few Real-Life Experiences from My Work*

In the following case studies, I will briefly illustrate how meditation and book psychotherapy intervention was used with my patients in Singapore.

My patient Mona (name disguised) was unable to forget her past and remembered all the pains of her past life. Mona is married with two daughters, ages 21 and 25. She had been in pain for four years and identified her past husband in this present life as a young Singaporean business tycoon. As her counsellor, I had to help her distinguish the past from the present. Using meditation and spiritual books, Mona was able to focus more clearly and began to relax and release the negative thoughts that contributed to her pain. Once she gained these insights, cognitive therapy was introduced to help Mona transform negative self-talk and focus on her desired goals.

Sera was a banker who had a 4-year-old son. She worked in Singapore and fell in love with her colleague Myrof, who was ten years younger. However, Myrof did not want to marry her or take responsibility for her son. My approach with Sera was to first introduce book psychotherapy, followed by cognitive and behavioural therapy. Over a month, the use of spiritual books helped to relieve Sera from her depression. Once she moved past her depression, she was better able to detach from her anger and begin to prioritize her goals in relation to herself and her son. Overall, these case studies show how meditation and book psychotherapy provide therapeutic measures for healing patients who are attempting to recover from traumas.

## 6—THE IMPORTANCE OF SEX EDUCATION

Sex education, in simple words, means 'being informed of human sexual behaviour, its reasons and implications'. Being aware of these helps an individual to be cautious and responsible. But what would be the perfect age to be informed? Should it be taught to an adolescent who has the option of being sexually active? Some argue that this might even encourage them to have sex. But as the old saying goes, 'It's better to be safe than sorry.'

*Why Is Sex Education Necessary?*

People are concerned that providing information about sex and sexuality arouses curiosity and can even lead to sexual experimentation. Contrary to that, studies have shown that sex education has not increased sexual activity. It has either reduced sexual activity or increased rates of condom use. It should, therefore, be provided to young people before the age of puberty and upwards before they establish their patterns of behaviour. The precise age should depend on the physical, emotional, and intellectual developments of the young people as well as their level of information.

It should be carefully delivered and at the right time. Sex is a basic human motivation. Parents should be more like friends during a child's puberty (the process of physical changes during which the child grows into adulthood and is capable of reproduction) and adolescent stage.

Sex is not a crime. The aim is to reduce risks of unwanted outcomes from risky sexual behaviour, which may lead to unwanted teenage pregnancies, sexual abuse, and contraction of a sexually transmitted infections, such as HIV, among other complications. Through sex education, youth learn and adopt the right attitudes towards sex. It helps youth have a positive mindset about sex and their sexuality. It helps to improve relationships between young people. It also empowers the youth against sexual abuse. Some psychologists believe that most personality defects are caused by sexual difficulties that remain repressed in areas of the mind. Sex is the root cause of many mental problems and might culminate into physical problems.

## Which Credible Sources Offer Sex Education for Children?

Some parents are open and feel comfortable discussing sex with their children, but that is not very common. In the Indian context, parents are often uncomfortable to provide sex education to their young ones. They believe sex education should be delivered in schools or by healthcare providers. In such cases, contributions from reliable external sources, like religious leaders, media, magazines, and sex education websites, could prove helpful in providing the right guidance beyond what a competent teacher can offer.

In most Western schools, sex education is taught as part of health and wellness modules, in junior high school or high school. Subjects like biology also educate students about the reproductive systems, male and female anatomy, and other relevant facts, such as menstruation, physical and emotional changes of adolescence, pregnancy, and contraception. Even subjects like home economics, physical education, and moral science can teach a child about practical issues such as sexual violence, homosexuality, sexually transmitted infections (STIs), safe sex, resisting peer pressure, sexual abuse, and even teenage pregnancies.

However, not all schools offer sex education, and it still remains a controversial issue in several countries due to religious stigma, social stigma, and local laws. In India, attempts by state governments to introduce sex education as a compulsory part of school curriculum have often been met with harsh criticism by people who claim it is against Indian culture and would mislead children.

## 7—DEALING WITH MARRIAGE WOES

Dealing with a failed or failing marriage can be a traumatic experience. The role of a marriage counsellor is crucial to restoring faith in such situations. In this article, we take a closer look at the art of new-age marriage counselling.

A marriage prospers when there is a good relationship between husband and wife. It is paramount that they understand each other's likes and dislikes, and there should be a strong emotional bond between them. Whether married or in a committed relationship, either partner has to be careful of the similarities and differences of the other, and an acceptance of the differences is crucial to sustain the relationship. To understand your partner, one of the best practices is to write down a list of his or her qualities, attitudes, skills, and interests so that you can appreciate your partner better.

Doing this exercise separately and then doing it together can help resolve conflict, increase intimacy, and improve communication skills between couples. My approach to relationship counselling is focussed on the present and future direction. I integrate the theories and therapies of counselling to bring about improvements in a short period of time within four to six sessions.

Most common problems encountered by couples who require counselling include interpersonal communication issues, differences in perspectives leading to heated arguments and disharmony, anger management, sexual incompatibility, emotional unhappiness, and lack of love in the relationship.

Continued dissatisfaction due to any of the above factors is a chief cause of extramarital affairs. In such situations, I try to establish a new platform to build trust and attempt to engage the suffering couples in building a new relationship ensuring effective measures against stress and anxiety.

## Premarriage and Postmarriage Counselling

In earlier times, most marriages took place when the couples were in their midtwenties. Adjustments to each other might have been easier. Nowadays, with late marriages, the partners are likely to be more diverse, and differences can be many and sometimes difficult to reconcile. Thus premarriage counselling becomes important to bring awareness of new roles and responsibilities. Premarriage counselling can also reduce postmarital problems. Couples are helped to prepare for a successful marriage and ensure a good chemistry sparks off before they get married.

## Is Not Having Children in a Family Any Cause for Disharmony?

Failure to conceive a baby can be very painful, especially if the childless couple is surrounded by families with children. They watch their friends give birth to two or three children and suffer the deprivation of the joy that a child brings into someone's life. They feel the emptiness of not being able to experience the same joy. The infertile spouse may feel guilty or inferior to the partner, and this can strain their married life.

### Do You Also Involve the Family for Marriage Counselling?

Family counselling is required only if it can be used to reinforce trust. Reality therapy teaches couples how to manage wants and needs in a relationship. It can help a couple to face the realities of situations in order to restore harmony in their marriage.

### What Is the Importance of a Healthy Sexual Life in Marriage?

I would focus on improving the sexual relationship by reflecting on intimacy, which ultimately relieves stress in a relationship. Talking about lovemaking and one's likes and dislikes go a long way towards making married sex life enjoyable. A fulfilling sex life means recognising the need for flexibility and changeability, and that the needs are different on different occasions. Just as our appetite for food varies—occasionally, we might want an elaborate three-course meal, which involves planning and preparation, while at other times, we might want a quick snack or a sandwich on the run—similarly, our sexual appetite varies, and variety maintains interest.

### How to Improve a Sexual Relationship

Communicate well, talk to your partner while making love, and be flexible. Focus on the sensation, spend some time just touching and stroking each other. Overcome the inhibitions: for example, if you have deeply ingrained beliefs that sex is 'dirty', sinful, or should not be pleasurable, try to reexamine your attitudes. Make time and create a special atmosphere with soft music, lights, and candles. It is important to figure out what is most important to each individual and create a unified view as a couple. These are lifelong skills to a successful marriage, time management, family/work priorities, and family time.

## 9—IMPROVING SELF-PROJECTION SKILLS

*What Sort of Engagements Influence Personalities Positively?*

One must identify the talents which lie dormant in the self. For example, you may be good at creative arts like dance, painting, music, or any other form which enhances self-recognition and self-esteem. During childhood, it is the parents' duty to look out for these seeds and provide nourishment, training, and encouragement to a personality. Later in life, one has to pursue these interests on his or her own.

Self-projection is considered one of the most profound and subtle ways of human psychological processes and is extremely difficult to work with. This is because the skills backing this process are hidden. It's creative only when projected to the outside world. Improving self-projection reduces anxiety by allowing an expression to these creative and unconscious impulses or desires without the conscious mind recognising them.

A creative process can be a health-enhancing and growth-producing experience. It has great value in improving projection because it doesn't resist inquiry into the truth. We also tend to confuse the concepts of intelligence and creativity as being the same thing, but they are quite different. Intelligence is the global capacity of an individual to act purposefully, think rationally, and deal effectively in the context of his or her environment. Creativity, on the other hand, is a mental process involving the generation of new ideas or concepts, or new associations between existing ideas or concepts.

Art is a means of symbolic communication. It is referred to as art psychotherapy, which emphasises the elements, such as drawings, paintings, and other artistic expressions, as being helpful in communicating issues, emotions, and resolving internal conflicts. From an artist's perspective, indulgence in art is seen as an opportunity to express oneself imaginatively, authentically, and spontaneously. It is considered to be an experience that, over time, can lead to personal fulfilment, emotional reparation, and transformation. Use of art helps to increase insight and judgment, allowing one to cope better with stress, work through traumatic experiences, and improve relationships with family and friends.

## Dance Therapy

Dance is a more appealing form of self-projection which works as a therapy. Dance therapy, or dance movement therapy (DMT), was founded on the basis of movement and emotion, on rhythm, sound, and vibrations. The ultimate purpose of DMT is to deliver a healthy balance and a sense of wholeness.

DMT strengthens the body-and-mind connection through body movements and improves both the mental and physical well-being of individuals. This therapy is also an effective aid in healing other disabilities and diseases, such as autism and learning disabilities.

DMT enhances organisational skills, mental capabilities of control and choice, and self-confidence. DMT has worked well in improving body image, social skills, coordination, and promoting communication. It reduces the feelings of isolation and provides inspiration for relationships in deaf and hearing-impaired persons. Dance also works for the blind and physically handicapped by improving their body image, motor skills, and personal awareness. Among the elderly too, DMT provides social interaction, expression, and exercise; alleviates fears of loneliness and isolation; and addresses eating disorders.

## Yoga Therapy

Yoga therapy involves self-expression based on Indian mythology. The best projections are of Lord Shiva in various forms of yoga and dances depicting his moods. Ancient Vedic scriptures have given vigorous combinations of yoga and dance to achieve positive mental health, which is the joyful union of mind and body. Dance and yoga have long been described as two rivers stemming from the same source. In the simplest definitions, yoga and dance can be reduced to breathing with movement, or breath-guided movement. One major factor that links dance and yoga is the concept of prana, or the life force that stems from breath. The yogi and the dancer, however, have a closer relationship with prana and their own breathing habits. The major difference between yoga and dance is the focus. While we do yoga from a place inside the body and mind, and that's where the focus should stay throughout practice, it's never about achieving the 'perfect pose' or wanting to force the body into an asana or a particular posture. Dance, on the other hand, has its focus on outward performance and aesthetics.

*Is There Any Structured Way to Know One's Self-Concept Deficiencies, Thus Improving Self-Projection?*

Yes. The thematic apperception test (TAT) is what helps you to assess this. Sigmund Freud (1856–1939), the originator of psychoanalysis, used this test to evaluate a person's expression of thought, attitudes, observational capacity, and emotional responses to ambiguous test materials. In TAT, the ambiguous materials consist of a set of cards that portray human figures in a variety of settings and situations. The TAT is an example of a projective instrument, and it asks the subject to project his or her habitual patterns of thoughts and emotional responses onto the pictures on the cards. As people taking TAT proceed through the various story cards and tell stories about the pictures, they reveal their expectations from their relationships with peers, parents, or other authority figures, subordinates, and possible romantic partners. It is considered to be effective in eliciting information about a person's view of the world and his or her attitudes towards self and others. In addition to assessing the content of the stories that the subject is telling, the examiner also evaluates the subject's manner, vocal tone, posture, hesitations, and other signs of an emotional response to a particular story picture. Many psychologists prefer not to call it a 'test'.

*How Do I Practise Self-Projection Skills in Daily Life?*

The above-mentioned test requires the ability to receive, process, and use feedback coming from within the 'self', outside of self, and the interaction between self and others. This generates a response which becomes feedback by the use of body, emotions, feelings, thoughts, and actions. It also enables listening to your body sensations, going inward and concentrating on every impulse of the body.

## 10—SWIM THERAPY

While swimming, one can learn to release tensions created by shocks and traumas of daily living. It helps to build a healthy digestive system, strengthen abdominal muscles, and improve posture. Breathing exercises in water help to relax the mind and also strengthen the lungs and improve stamina. For elderly people, swimming is a good therapy to build healthy joints against joint pains.

Swimming and diving have been used successfully to treat phobia of heights if the problem is caused by dysfunction in maintaining body balance. This is quite important for people living and working in high-rise buildings in Singapore.

Speaking of phobias, which can prevent us from achieving our full potential, let's look at some very basic information about phobias and how swimming and aquatic exercise can help us overcome them. The phobia can be of a specific or social nature.

### What Are the Characteristics of a Specific Phobia?

A specific object or situation may trigger an intense fear which is out of proportion to what evokes it. The person recognises that it is unreasonable and irrational but cannot do anything about it. It interferes with the smooth functioning of everyday life. Avoiding the situation that creates the phobia is the normal strategy but is not a long-term solution. Examples of specific phobias are fear of bathing, insects, darkness, bridges, fire, airsickness, pain, wild animals, heights, dust, amnesia, wind, and driving a car.

### What Are the Characteristics of a Social Phobia?

A socially phobic person often worries about his or her social situation, focuses inward, begins to avoid company, loses confidence, and then worries and avoids more. Overestimating the negative evaluation that other people will make, social phobics often have one set of rules for themselves and one for others. This can lead to intense anxiety, panic attacks, and excessive anger. Examples of social phobias are fear of people, crowds, company, loneliness, newness, novelty, being laughed at, speaking in public, being touched, loud sounds, smiles, failure, and so on.

### Is There a Treatment for Phobia?

It helps to understand the process, mental framework, and factors sustaining the phobia. The therapist has to construct a desensitisation hierarchy technique and create a therapeutic situation.

The golden rule ultimately to overcome a phobia is to face it directly. Stay in the situation of fear until you notice your anxiety cooling down. Gaining some control over physical reactions of fear and anxiety, through relaxation training, breathing exercises, distraction, and positive talk helps.

## Can Swimming Be a Therapy to Counter Phobias?

Yes! It is not merely an exercise or a fun activity but has therapeutic applications too. For children (and adults too), it can remove inherent phobias and also help them develop resilience against tough emotional and physical conditions.

## How Can Swim Therapy Help?

The first step against phobias is to empower the person with the confidence to believe that whatever the phobia, it can be overcome. You can now take back your freedom and your life. One proven approach for confidence-building is through swim therapy, especially if the person is a nonswimmer or has fear of water (aquaphobia) or even fear of bathing (ablutophobia). It can be fast and permanent, and the best part is that no medicine is involved!

People will not like swim therapy if they are afraid of water. Such people can be desensitised to the fear of water if they take a bath regularly. Psychotherapists may initiate therapy in a shallow pool, then proceed to an invigorating Jacuzzi, before implementing swimming as an exercise and as therapy, using each stage to add to the client's confidence.

In therapy, for example, the client could be asked to imagine a big spider in the pool and touch it. Why a spider? Now, most of us might feel threatened by approaching creepy-crawlies, especially when we are struggling in water. Yet, we can learn from the tenacity of the spider that persistently weaves its web even after failing a number of times. Each time the failure reinforces its determination. Likewise, one can unwaveringly and positively work on one's phobia, step by step.

A swimming pool is an excellent location where the swimmer goes through these steps and trains his or her mind every moment. For a swimmer in therapy, every stroke is a choice between going ahead and sinking. As the swimmer becomes deft in moving ahead, overcoming fear becomes a habit which moulds his or her character and finally makes the person succeed in all adverse situations against any phobia.

## 11– BIPOLAR DISORDER

The cycle of moods from one extreme to another without any control is broadly termed as bipolar disorder. The experience can be of long periods of excitement ('high' or manic phase) and of being extremely depressed ('low' or depressive phase). In other words, bipolar disorder can be described as a roller coaster of emotions. Cycling can be rapid or slow. It has been found by researchers that people with bipolar disorder are of the slow-cycling type. They experience long periods of being up 'high' (manic phase) and of being down 'low' (depressive phase).

Bipolar disorder is also called 'manic depression'. A person with bipolar disorder experiences alternating 'highs'—what we clinicians call 'mania'—characterised by extreme happiness and hyperactivity. The slow-cycling type is known as depression and is characterised by extreme sadness, lack of energy, and inability to enjoy mental happiness. This change can be seen from a few hours to few days, or longer, lasting up to several weeks or even months.

Bipolar episodes can lead to many conflicts in everyday life, which can be challenging in maintaining a regular lifestyle. It becomes all the more difficult when the person appears to behave erratically and irresponsibly without any reason. Severe change of energy levels in body and mind of such a person in everyday life results in damage to human relationships, poor job performance, and low social self-esteem, all of which feed back into increasing the disorder.

## What Are the Contributing Factors of Bipolar Disorder?

The cause of bipolar disorder can be genetic, as studies have suggested that chromosomal as well as environmental conditions aggravate the disease. Recent life events and interpersonal relationships contribute to the onset and recurrences of bipolar mood episodes. Abnormalities in behaviour are reported by the family members, friends, and co-workers, followed by experts like psychiatrists and clinical psychologists.

## How Can We Treat Bipolar Disorder?

It can be controlled by a combination of medicine and psychotherapy. Psychotherapy is aimed at alleviating core symptoms, recognising episode triggers, and reducing negative emotions in relationships. Psychotherapy improves mental health and treats psychological disorders, facilitates the resolution of interpersonal conflicts, improves memory, reduces stress, and helps rationalise difficult issues related to everyday life.

I use psychotherapy as a scientific integrated model, drawing on the strengths of different approaches for my patients. Paying special attention to trust-building between the therapist and client is the key factor for a seamless transition from the current to the desired state. Foster a therapeutic relationship by providing an honest, open, and nonjudge mental contexts for clients to explore their issues and improve.

Paper-pencil questionnaires are routinely used to track progress towards therapy goals objectively and to ensure that the client is progressing. Practise cognitive behavioural therapy, family-focussed therapy, and psychodynamic therapy in modifying and healing. These approaches have been very efficient in preventing relapse and curing the disorder.

*What Are the Challenges and Rewards You See in Dealing with Your Patients?*

The acute phase is challenging because the patients show anger during counselling. It becomes a challenge for me to calm down and turn their red eyes normal. It takes a few sittings over a few months before the patient realises the benefits, and the reward is high satisfaction when I contribute to someone's life and happiness.

## 12—EMOTIONAL EXPLOSION

*How Do We Avoid an 'Emotional Explosion' or Outburst?*

We can learn to spot negative thoughts as they come up and then challenge them. Observing yourself and your behaviour as an objective third person is very helpful. An emotional flare-up can be a result of ongoing interactions amongst the following factors:

1. *Biological factors*: genes and current biological state.
2. *Psychological factors*: cognitions (thoughts and schemas), affect (feelings and moods), and overt behaviours.
3. *Social factors*: immediate social environment and culture.

Experiments have shown that we can learn techniques to overcome these negative emotions, manage ourselves out of these states of mind, and thus avoid emotional explosions such as fits of rage, depression, fear, jealousy, and envy. Address the explosion as soon as it arises. Timing is critical. In fact, the best thing to do is to catch the emotion the moment it occurs, then analyse its cause before rectifying it.

Take a break. Every excited person needs 'calming down'. Question yourself for the real reason for the explosions. The reasons for anger, disappointments, envy, and jealousy are often deeper than you might imagine. Redefine the problem from a new angle.

*How to Develop and Manage Cognitive Thinking*

For many people, challenging and changing with logic and evidence may be sufficient. But to achieve the best results in developing your cognitive thinking, a more systematic approach helps. It includes keeping a diary of significant events and associated feelings, thoughts, and behaviours, and questioning and testing cognitions, assumptions, evaluations, and beliefs. The analyses of this record let the person reorient his or her behavioural responses.

Learn to step back and look at yourself and observe yourself in the mirror; register your emotional state and say to yourself, 'You are really jealous/upset/hurt/disappointed/irritated.' Try to feel your emotions as they occur. Listen to your body's signals attached to each emotion and make a note of them. For example, I clench my fists when I am angry, I tap my fingers when I am impatient, and I sweat when I am nervous. Identify your 'dynamic emotions' (i.e., the emotions which work against you), which are the most difficult to manage, and the ones which damage your self-esteem.

Register the situations, events, and people that trigger your dynamic and destructive emotions. Consider whether a surface feeling may be caused by some underlying deeper feeling. Experiences happening at the surface level may be the result of deeper feelings of fear, disappointment, and frustration, which may still remain after the anger disappears. Gradually begin confronting the activities that you earlier feared to face, and try out new ways of behaving and reacting to them.

Revaluate the way you have been thinking about yourself up until now. List some of the negative thoughts you have of yourself, and then try to reverse those thoughts 180 degrees into positive ones and see how this makes you feel.

Avoid comparing yourself to others. List your strengths, positive attributes, and accomplishments that you are proud of, and reflect on them when you deal with the emotional explosions.

How things have changed in the last few months! Meeting people socially and for work, shopping, travelling, partying – all the things which were part of 'normal' life have come to a halt. We are by ourselves most of the time whether working from home, studying or involved in any other activity. There are cities in total lockdown where even stepping outside of the house is challenging.

We are social animals; devoid of human company now - practicing social distancing. Economic impact aside there is a whole range of adjustments needed on the emotional front. There is fear for oneself and the family members (many of whom you can't even meet now), anxiety about the future particularly financial security, numbness from an overdose of negative news on TV and social media. Family members can start getting on each other's nerves with everyone at home all the time. Suddenly there is a lot of time on our hands which in itself in creating anxiety in many.

We are connected to everything and everybody, especially our phones but we are least connected with ourselves. Now there is an opportunity for self-discovery; it is as though nature has hit the reset button just for that. It is harder/impossible to meet friends these days, we can try to find the 'friend within'. We have no control over infections in the physical world, we do have the power to control what gets into our minds, we could and should take care our minds do not get infected with negativity – tough but doable.

Giving in to pessimism is easy, onus is upon each one of us to be determined to stay positive and to encourage those around us to be upbeat as well. Discover optimists and stay connected with them, positivity is infectious too.

*Stay positive, spread positivity and be safe.*

Sanjiv Aiyar
Founder CEO
ApKar Consulting Pte. Ltd., Singapore

Printed in the United States
By Bookmasters